AIR FRYER OVEN COOKBOOK

AMAZINGLY EASY AND QUICK AIR FRYER RECIPES

AUTHOR

Jack Rox

Table of contents

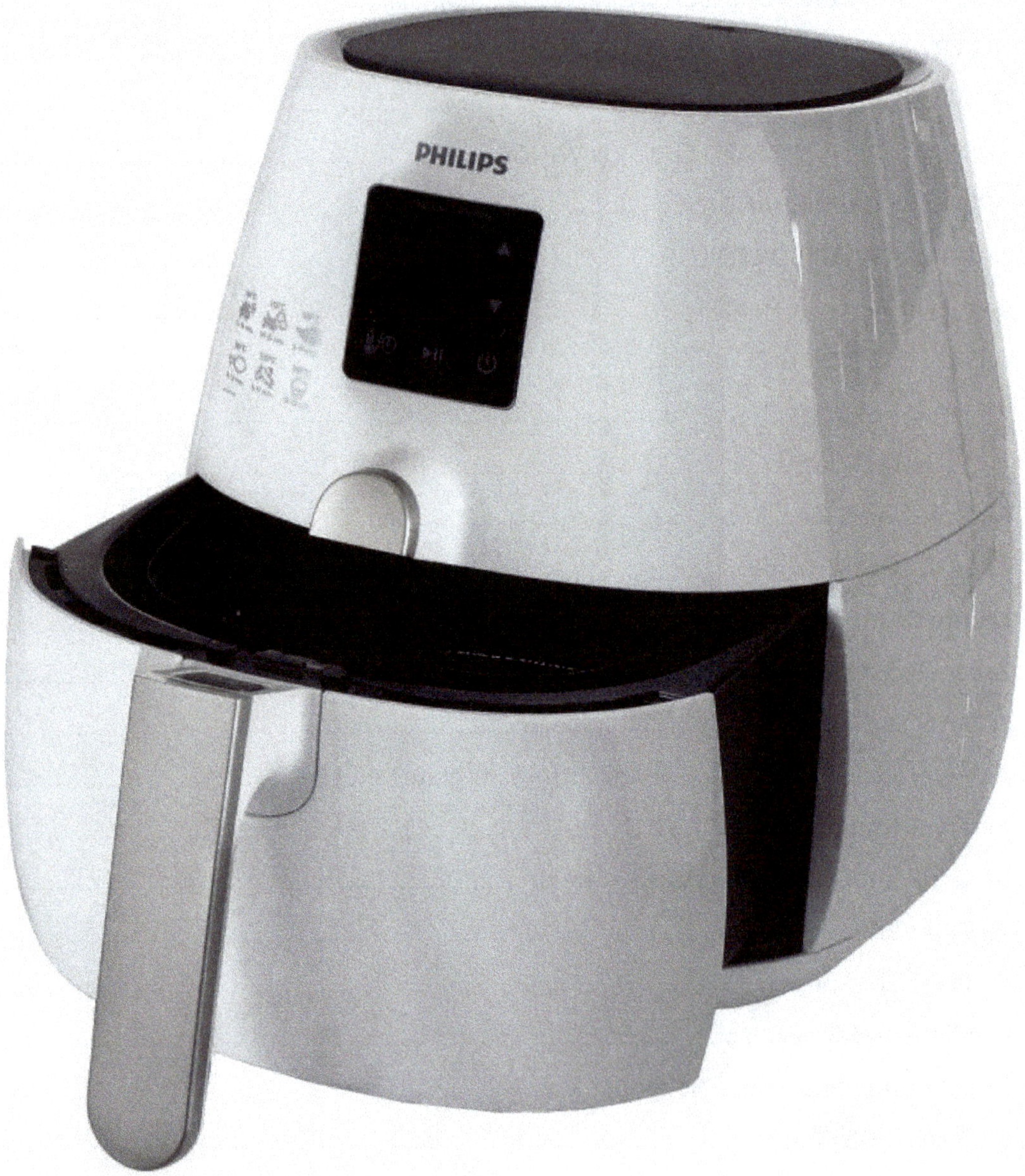
PHILIPS

AIR FRYER OVENCOOKBOOK

AMAZINGLY EASY AND QUICK AIR FREYER RECIPES TOFRY , ROAST AND BAKE DELICIOUS MEALS AND LOSE WEIGHT

INTRODUCTION TOAN AIR FRYER

An air fryer is an advanced kitchen machine that prepares nourishment by circling tourists around it as opposed to utilizing oil. It offers a low-fat adaptation of nourishments that would customarily be cooked in a profound fryer. Therefore, by and large, unfortunate nourishments, for example, French fries, singed chicken, and onion rings are cooked with no oil or up to 80 percent less fat substance contrasted with regular cooking strategies. The Air Fryer gives more advantageous singed nourishments and suppers, empowering you to be freed of the calories that accompany eating seared food sources while as yet giving you that crunchiness, surface, and quality that you want.

This family unit apparatus works by circling sight-seeing (up to 400°F) equitably and rapidly around nourishment fixing that is put in an encased space. The warmth makes the nourishment fixing fresh and dry outwardly, however delicate and soggy within. The air fryer can be utilized on essentially everything. Other than searing, you can flame broil, heat, and dish. Its assortment of cooking choices makes it simpler to prepare any sort of feast whenever of the day.

Air fryers are progressive kitchen apparatuses that utilization superheated air to broil nourishments. EIn any case, that is only the tip of the nourishment you can cook in your air fryer.

We love the flavor of Pan fried nourishments, yet not the calories or chaos. Air singing is an extraordinary method to cook nourishments quick, simple, and in less time. It warms up rapidly and courses tourist internally to prepare nourishment and consistently seal in all the normal juices. Air fryers permit you to broil, heat, flame broil, or steam nourishment is more advantageous, quicker, and all the more helpfully.

This formula book highlights breakfast, vegetables, sides, primary dishes, and even pastries! These are only a portion of the nourishment you will have the option to cook in your air fryer. This book will work with each size and style of the air fryer. You can likewise prepare them with enlistment air cooking. Let these plans motivate you to cook solid, well-adjusted suppers for you and your family.

THE AIR FRYER AND AIR FRYING?

Air fryers are fundamentally scaled-down ledge convection ovens with a heating component over the food and a solid fan. As it creates heat, the fan circles the sight-seeing to enable the food to cook equitably and crispy. When contrasted with customary rotisserie foods, most air fried food surfaces have fundamentally the same as smash without utilizing a huge amount of oil or fat. Truth be told, we scarcely need to utilize any oil and the food despite everything that turns out crispy and scrumptious. Most food likewise turns out like it's flawlessly roasted in a convection oven with magnificent roasted flavors and surfaces. When breaded and splashed with oil, food becomes crunchy and fundamentally the same as what you would cook in a profound fryer. For certain dishes like chicken wings, they cook incredibly fresh with no oil. Generally, food is crispy roasted and crunchy without all the fat. Past considering air fryers as a substitute for profound browning, consider them small scale convection ovens, and the entirety of the abrupt the potential outcomes become inestimable.

WHY AN AIR FRYER COOKBOOK?

We needed to tell everybody that air broiling isn't about re-heating solidified comfort foods. Indeed, it's incredible for heating remains and cooking snappy solidified bites. You can absolutely cook crisp, healthy, and healthy recipes in the air fryer. No doubt. Try not to JUDGE. Truly, we made a decision from the start, yet after our first straightforward feast for 2 individuals in under 20 minutes, we were snared and fixated and wild. Consequently, the formation of overly new and delightful recipes for the cookbooks.
Why Use It

Low-Fat Meals: Unarguably, the most basic advantage of the air fryer is its utilization of sight-seeing circulation to prepare nourishment fixings from all edges, in this manner wiping out the requirement for oil use. This makes it workable for individuals on a low-fat eating regimen to serenely prepare brilliantly sound suppers.

More beneficial Foods& Environment:: Air fryers are intended to work without swelling oils and to deliver more advantageous nourishments with up to 80 percent less fat. This makes it simpler to get in shape since you can at present eat your seared dishes while moderating the calories and soaked fat. Doing that change to a more advantageous life is increasingly reachable by utilizing this apparatus. Your house is additionally freed of the fragrance that accompanies Pan-fried nourishments that regularly remains around the climate even a few hours after profound broiling.

Multipurpose Use: The air fryer empowers you to perform various tasks as it can prepare numerous dishes on the double. It is yours across the board machine that can flame broil, heat, fry, and meal those dishes that you love! You never again need numerous apparatuses for different occupations. It can do different employments separate machines will do. It can barbecue meat, cook veggies, and heat baked goods. It fills in as a viable substitution for your broiler, profound fryer, and stovetop.

Incredibly Safe: Remember how extra cautious you must be while tossing chicken or some different fixings into the profound fryer? You need to guarantee that the hot oil doesn't spill and consume your skin since it's in every case extremely hot. With your air fryer, you wouldn't have to stress over brunt skin from hot oil spillage. It does all the broiling and is totally protected. By the by, use cooking gloves while repositioning your fryer to maintain a strategic distance from dangers from the warmth.

Furthermore, keep your air fryer out of youngsters' compass.

Simple Clean Up: The Air Fryer leaves no oil and, along these lines, no wreckage. Tidy up time is agreeable since their oils spill to clean on dividers and floors, and no rejecting or scouring of the container. The Air fryer parts are made of non-stick material, which keeps nourishment from adhering to surfaces along these lines, making it difficult to clean. These parts are anything but difficult to clean and keep up. They are removable and dishwasher-sheltered too.

Spare Valuable Time: People who are on tight calendars can utilize the quickness of the air fryer to make tasty suppers. For occasions, you can make French fries in under 15 minutes and heat a cake inside 25 minutes. Inside minutes as well, you can appreciate fresh chicken fingers or brilliant fries. On the off chance that you are consistently in a hurry, the air fryer is perfect for you since you will invest less energy in the kitchen. It empowers you to deal with your rushed and occupied day by day life, filling your heart with joy increasingly sensible.

Essential Parts, Accessories and Their Importance

Prepare your fixings and put it into the crate, and afterward set your clock. The tourist goes to work, and when its work is finished, the clock goes off with a ding sound, showing that your nourishment is finished. You may even check your nourishment to perceive how it's advancing without upsetting the set time. When you pull out the container, the fryer will delay; when you place back the skillet, warming will proceed.

The Airfryer is a direct apparatus, with no collecting required and no confusion. It comprises of three principle things; the cooking container, the skillet, and the primary fryer unit.

The Cooking Basket is the place you put your nourishment. It has a crate handle where you place your hand when taking care of the apparatus and prepared nourishment to forestall consumes or wounds when the air fryer is turned on. The bushel fits splendidly into the skillet. The Pan gathers the nourishment remainders and overabundance oil and fits impeccably into the airfryer& then we have The Main Fryer Unit, which comprises numerous parts. There are other helpful parts that incorporate rack, twofold flame broil layer, a bushel, and nourishment separators that make it conceivable to prepare various dishes immediately.

Tips For Usage

Keep It Dry: Pat dry nourishments before cooking, particularly marinated nourishments. Doing this will forestall overabundance smoke and splattering. Nourishments that contain high-fat substances, for example, chicken bosom and wings, for the most part, store fat when cooking. Therefore, ensure you void the kept fat from the base of the air fryer on occasion.

Space Your Foods: Overcrowding is a no-no with the air fryer. In the event that you need your nourishments to cook well, give it a lot of room with the goal that air can flow well. You need to appreciate the firmness of your dinners, isn't that so? Congestion keeps air from coursing over the nourishments. So make certain to space nourishments out.

Shake Foods Around: Open the Air Fryer at regular intervals of cooking and shake around nourishments in the bin. Chips, French fries, and other littler nourishments can pack, however, shaking around forestalls that. Pivot nourishments each 5 to 10 minutes to empower them to cook and shape well.

Splash Foods. You will require your cooking splash when utilizing your air fryer as it assists with keeping nourishments from adhering to the bin. Shower nourishments gently, or you could simply include a smidgen of oil.

Cook in Batches: The air fryer has a little cooking limit. IOn the off chance that you are cooking for countless individuals, you should cook in clumps.

Preheat air fryer when it has not been utilized for some time. Preheat for 3-5 minutes to permit it to heat up appropriately.

Presently you can utilize your air fryer to prepare the painstakingly chose sound and scrumptious plans beneath. Just adhere to the directions and appreciate balanced dinners for you and your family.

INSTRUCTIONS TO COOK HEALTHY FOOD WITH AIR FRYER

It's anything but difficult to cook healthy air fried foods since you don't require as a lot of oil. The hot flowing heat crisps and roasts food superbly without the requirement for a great deal of oil. So generally speaking, yes, air fried food can be healthier. Segment control is another significant factor, and on the off chance that you eat more than the one suggested serving, you've quite recently blown the "healthy" out of air singing. Air singing is only one method to cook healthier food. The amount you eat is clearly significant as well!

PROS AND WHY WE LOVE AIR FRYING:

- Perfect for two individuals or littler segments. For multiple individuals, there's such a significant number of greater models out there to cook bigger parts. The potential outcomes are inestimable.

- It's a healthier method of cooking fried or crispy foods. In general, you can utilize substantially less oil to accomplish crunchy and crispy finished foods.
- The kind of food is brilliant in light of the fact that the heat gives a pleasantly fresh and "burn."
- There's tidy little up and less splattering of oil while cooking. Everything gets contained pleasantly inside the air fryer while cooking.
- Food cooks fresh due to the littler cooking zone, and the heating component is nearer to the food.
- Because of littler bins, the food cooked speedier when contrasted with ovens and no pre-heating is fundamental.
- You don't need to heat up your home in Summer when you're longing for something warm, roasted or pan-fried
- Great for cooking solidified foods without oil and extraordinary or pre-heating foods.

THE CONS AND WHY IT MIGHT NOT BE FOR YOU:

• You truly can't cook enormous servings of food except if you purchase the bigger air fryers. Purchasing bigger air fryers is a major venture and except if you use it enough.

• If you need to cook a great deal of food from the little air fryer, you will need to cook in bunches. That will take heaps of time sitting tight for one dish to cook before you start the following one.

• They aren't too modest, and some can be more problematic to clean, contingent upon the plan and model. A few models are extraordinary and make tidy up excessively simple. Anyway, different models are somewhat more work to clean.

• You ought to have great ventilation in your kitchen in light of the fact that the hot fast cooking discharges bunches of sight-seeing. A few foods like bacon and chicken thighs may smoke in view of the high-fat substance. There are approaches to cure the smoking as well.

• If you, as of now, have a little ledge convection oven and love it, you should adhere to that, except if you're into extremely overly low oil cooking.
and garlic powder

FUNDAMENTAL INSTRUCTIONS TO NOTE WHEN COOKING AIR FRIED FOODS:

- Don't stuff the crates with food. Cook in bunches on the off chance that you have to (2 little, medium clusters cook superior to 1 enormous clump).
- Don't neglect to shake while cooking, yet in some cases shaking the crate during cooking isn't sufficient. Tenderly hurl the food with an elastic spatula, so food doesn't break or tear.
- The base of the air fryers can get hot while cooking. Make a point to put on a heat-safe surface or lush cutting board.
- Avoid utilizing the high fuel cooking showers since they can cause the inside coating of non-stick containers to strip. Continuously use spritzer or siphon-style oil splashes. In addition, it generally tastes better when you can utilize genuine olive oil or quality cooking oil. You can purchase extraordinary siphons to add your oil too.

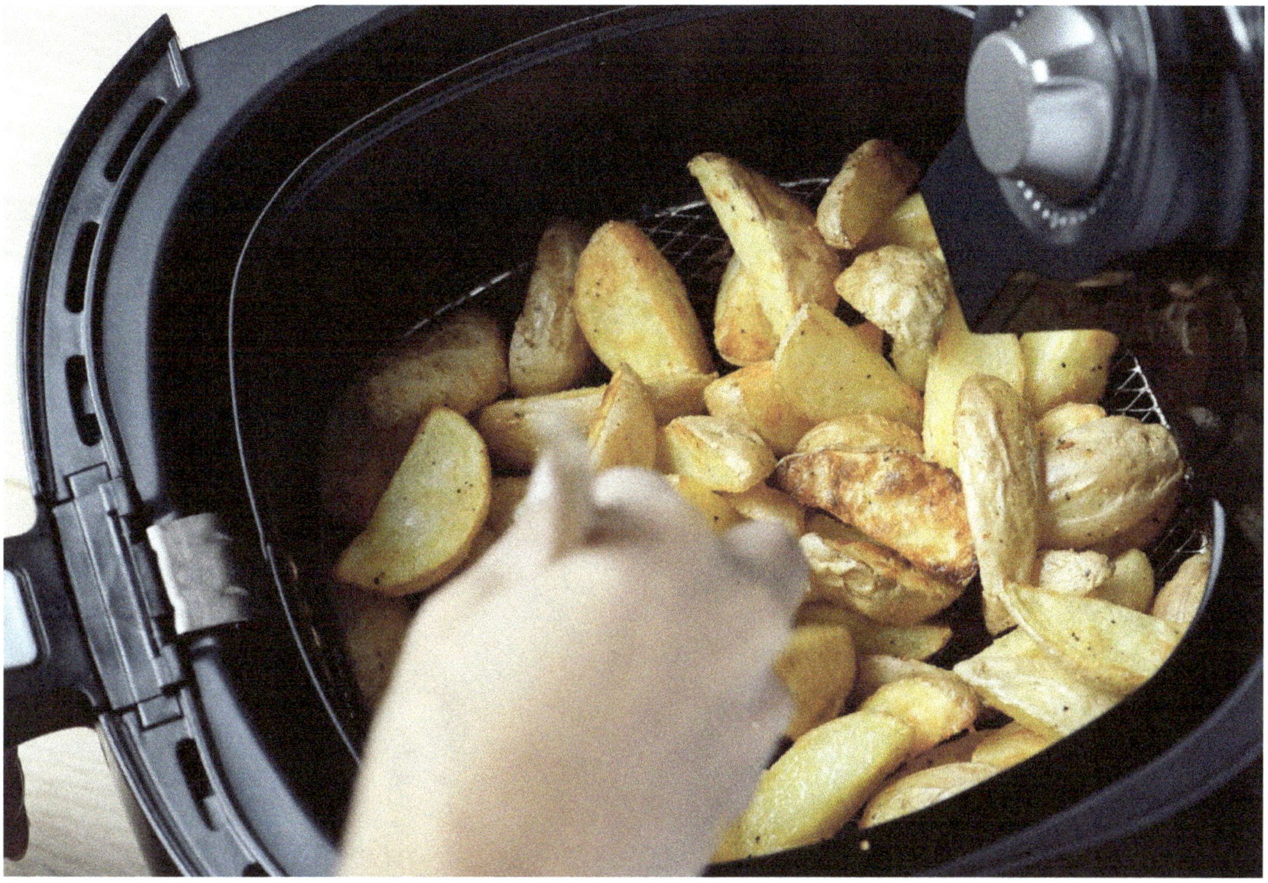

THE BEST TYPE OF AIR FRYER

There are various kinds of air fryers, every single diverse brand, and with various top picks.

- Size matters, particularly in case you're expecting to sustain a group of four to six hungry individuals.
- We're for the most part cooking for two during the bustling weeknights, and the 3 qt size fryers are extraordinary for us.
- If you're thinking about what size of air fryer to get our proposal is the 3-4 qt sizes for 2-3 individuals (or if its all the same to you cooking numerous bunches) and the 5-6 qt for groups of 4-6 (you'll despite everything cook somethings in clumps, yet not as much as the littler air fryers).

Here are the best air fryers positioned, all together:

1. Philips Airfryer XXL
2. Cuisinart Compact AirFryer
3. Cuisinart Airfryer Toaster Oven
4. Ninja Air Fryer
5. Ninja Foodi
6. Dash Compact Air Fryer
7. Breville Smart Oven Air
8. GoWise 8-in-1 Air Fryer XL 5.9 Qt.
9. Krups Easy Fry Deluxe Digital Air Fryer 4.2 L
10. Farberware 3.2-Quart Digital Oil-Less Fryer
11. Black and Decker Crisp 'N Bake Air Fry Toaster Oven
12. Krups Fry Delight
13. Power Air Fryer XL

14. Black and Decker 2L Purifry Air Fryer

15. Instant Vortex Plus Air Fryer Oven

16. NuWave Brio Digital Air Fryer 6 Quart

17. NuWave Bravo XL Smart Oven

18. Oster DuraCeramic Air Fryer

Philips Airfryer XXL

With regards to searing, the Philips Airfryer XXL is the best air fryer we tried and the easiest to use. During testing, I tasted a dreadful parcel of French fries, and it cooked up the ones I was unable to quit noshing on. They had the combo of crunchiness, delicacy, and potato enhance that make incredible fries so luscious. In any event, when I stacked the bushel with multiple pounds of solidified fries, they turned out crispy. Battered Nashville hot chicken turned out with a snapping covering as though it had been rotisserie, and burgers equaled ones made on the barbecue with the Philips Airfryer.

Presently, this is a major, overwhelming, and extravagant machine that is noisier than most when it's working. It doesn't have computerized controls, and hence it's difficult to set the temperature and clock accurately. With a couple of a bigger number of parts than most air fryers, there's a whole other world to clean, and keeping in mind that the entirety of the parts can go in the dishwasher, the tremendous bin will eat up considerable retire and counter space. Similar to all air fryers, it's still generally simple to utilize—this one requires no preheat—and the outcomes merit the result. A simple to peruse formula book is incorporated to give you heaps of thoughts.

What settles on the Philips Airfryer, our top decision is that it's consistently the absolute best at air searing, even with huge family-size parts of healthier fried foods. Also, you can detect that for heaps of cash, and you're getting a strong, well-constructed machine. In the event that you cook for a recognizing group that truly prefers fried food yet not the fat, I think Philips is certainly worth the venture.

Pros

• Huge limit

• No preheat required

• Foods turn out crispy.

Cons

• Expensive

• Takes up a great deal of room

• Noisy and Heavy

Cuisinart Compact AirFryer

The primary thing you'll see about the Cuisinart Compact AirFryer is that not normal for most air fryers, it's not strangely molded like a gigantic egg or space case. Or maybe it's a major tempered steel block that resembles a shortened toaster oven. While its square-shaped shape causes it to fit all the more conveniently on a ledge or in a cupboard, the Cuisinart, despite everything takes up a touch of ledge land (regardless of its name).

You'll discover that Cuisinart is a moderately uncomplicated apparatus as far as heating components. It doesn't have preset cooking projects for explicit foods or extra capacities like "keep warm" or get dried out, to make the cooking procedure simpler. You basically go dials to set the temperature and the cooking time, and there's no compelling reason to preheat. There's additionally a straight forward manual that incorporates recipes to kick you off on air browning.

Since it has a wide bushel, food can be spread out to get all the more even and crispy outcomes with moderately brisk cooking times without the food drying out in the time it takes to air fry. Most other air fryers constrain you to heap the food over one another, which can make lopsided outcomes. Utilizing the Cuisinart Compact AirFryer, custom made fries looked and had an aftertaste like they had been weaving in a profound fryer tank of oil.

Neither the treated steel container nor the trickle skillet is dishwasher safe, so it's not really simple to clean. At the point when you cook drippy battered things like tempura shrimp or onion rings, you may need to utilize a little exertion to get them unblemished. Notwithstanding, in case you're searching for an apparatus to air broil and do it well, and would prefer not to pay an extravagant sum, this Cuisinart is definitely justified even despite your consideration.

Pros

• Uncomplicated to program

• Doesn't require preheating

• Foods turn out crispy.

• Helpful manual

Cons

• Controls aren't computerized

• Parts are not dishwasher sheltered or nonstick.

BEST MULTIPURPOSE AIR FRYER

Cuisinart Air Fryer Toaster Oven

While not modest, the Cuisinart Airfryer Toaster Oven is certainly less expensive, also more space-productive, than purchasing two generally enormous ledge apparatuses. It accompanies an air fryer container to be utilized alongside an air fryer setting. I thought that it was filled in also, and sometimes, its heat component was superior to air fryers at carmelizing and crisping. What's more, it toasted incredibly equitably.

In contrast to most models in this value classification, it doesn't have computerized controls. While it is anything but an enormous machine, it is taller than regular toaster ovens. It suits 2 pounds of fries, 6 cuts of bread and as per Cuisinart, a 4-pound chicken. In the event that you love to hurl everything in the dishwasher, know that every one of the parts should be cleaned by hand. In any case, except if you as of now have a toaster oven that you love, the Cuisinart is a decent purchase for its adaptability.

Pros

• It's a toaster, ledge oven, and air fryer.

• Foods turn out crispy.

• Toasts uniformly

Cons

• Controls aren't advanced.

• Parts aren't nonstick.

• Not dishwasher safe

How Does an Air Fryer Work?

First of all, air fryers are not really fryers, but instead ledge convection ovens that course is sight-seeing around foods in a bin. Utilizing all things considered a half tablespoon of oil, they unquestionably darker and fresh up food; however, not as equally as browning. What's more, things don't generally turn out with a similar mix of all-over crunchiness and ideal delicacy as they do when they're dropped in hot oil. In any case, air fryers don't require in excess of a couple of moments to preheat, which implies through and through they convey the products quicker than profound or oven-broiling. Additionally, I found they didn't radiate any cooking scents, so your home never possesses a scent like a chicken shack.

The best air fryers can likewise be utilized as an oven to cook meats, meals, or even heated merchandise. They are, obviously, restricted by their size and don't offer any bit of leeway here over a conventional oven.Be that as it may, If you utilize your oven for capacity, it will, in general, heat up the kitchen, or you frequently wish you had an additional oven, an air fryer can prove to be useful. One thing to know: These kitchen instruments are large and strangely formed, so they take up a great deal of ledge space and aren't anything but difficult to store.

Primary concern: If you find crispy foods compelling yet need to maintain a strategic distance from the fat, an air fryer may be exactly what you're searching for.

What Cooks Best In An Air Fryer?

It relies upon how inventive you can get! Meats, vegetables, and even prepared merchandise can work in your air fryer. Also, there are huge amounts of air fryer formula books available at this point.

Some famous alternatives include:

• Vegetables, for example, potatoes, carrots, squash—basically anything you would roast on a preparing sheet

• Meat dishes, for example, breaded chicken, battered chicken, bacon, burgers, and sausages.

• Frozen foods like chicken chunks, mozzarella sticks, onion rings, and french fries

• Baked products, for example, doughnuts, wastes, and pipe cake.

Air-Frying Tips

Assessed cooking staff author Valerie Li offers this air-browning guidance:

• Preheat the air fryer before cooking. Since an air fryer is fundamentally a smaller convection oven, the preheating stage can help keep food from over-cooking. When all is said in done, preheat at 375°F for three to five minutes, contingent upon the size of the fryer.

• Use heating powder on the off chance that you are making chicken wings. By covering the wings in preparing powder, the peptide bond in chicken skin will separate because of an expansion in the pH level. This will allow the chicken skin to get crispy and dark-colored.

• Lay all food as level as would be prudent. An excessively packed singing crate can prompt unevenly fried foods, and undesirable consumes. Maintain a strategic distance from this, ensure you separate the food and cook just little groups one after another. This is particularly significant in case you're heating solidified fries—the water can make them wet!

• Frying bland food produces acrylamide. One regular approach to diminish starch content is to whiten fixings before cooking.

Other Air Fryers We Tested

Ninja Air Fryer

The Ninja Air Fryer gave our top of the line Philips Airfryer XXL a run for the cash. You could have persuaded me that both breaded and battered chicken pieces were fried in the best solid metal skillet. French fries approached the genuine article yet didn't have an incredible allover crunch that you get from a fryer or the Philips (which can get even fresh up an entire pack of French fries without a moment's delay). In any case, the Ninja is about a fourth of the cost of the Philips and is not even close as large or overwhelming.

On the Ninja, you'll find computerized controls and settings for reheating, roasting, and drying out. More alternatives make for progressively confused programming, yet after a couple of cooks, you'll effectively ace the important advances. The nonstick covered crate can be hurled in the dishwasher. With this air fryer, you likewise get a hardened steel rack for staggered cooking.

Pros

• An air fryer and multi-cooker in one

• Digital controls

• Food turns out crispy.

Cons

• Very huge and substantial

• Cookbook not accommodating

• Noisy

Ninja Foodi

I confess to having had a healthy portion of incredulity when it went to the Ninja Foodi, an apparatus that notwithstanding being an air fryer, is additionally a pressure cooker and a slow cooker. All things considered, I'm here to reveal to you that it not exclusively does both, it does them both well. Indeed, it cooked the crunchiest, and most well-sautéed brings about our air fryer cook-off, in addition to its pressures cooks just as any I've at any point tried (Reviewed named it the best overhaul pick in the best pressure cookers manage, as well).

On the off chance that you like, you can even consolidate the two capacities, pressure cooking a chicken and afterward sautéing and crisping the skin reporting in real-time fry setting. Extra projects on the Foodi allow you to sear, get dried out, steam, slow cook, and sauté, making it the most adaptable multicooker available. One thing significant: During air fricasseeing mode, it's noisier than most.

IAs you would expect with such huge numbers of choices, it takes a little practice to get the hang of programming the computerized controls. Notwithstanding, the screen is all around planned with huge simple to understand lettering. The Food is space-sparing contrasted with owning both an air fryer and a multi-cooker, yet it is a huge, substantial machine that you won't have any desire to lift all through a bureau. It merits giving it a devoted spot on a ledge in the event that you intend to exploit its flexibility and use it regularly. Considering the multi-usefulness of this machine, I wish the cookbook that accompanies it was better sorted out and had recipes and graphs for the entirety of the capacities. The container and the pot are nonstick covered and alright for dishwasher cleaning. However, the tops require TLC.

Pros

• Cooks well overall

• Includes air fryer work

• Versatile

Cons

• Expensive

• Oversized

Run Compact Air Fryer

This little person is simply so darn charming you can't resist cherishing (It's likely why such a significant number of Amazon analysts go gaga for this air fryer). The Dash Compact Air Fryer makes an OK showing of "browning" as long as you bind it to about a half-pound of food at once. No preheating is required; however, for the best outcomes, you have to hurl or turn things a couple of times during cooking.

With its dial controls, you can't set the Dash exactly. Generally, the manual is useful and even incorporates a couple of recipes, yet a portion of the temperatures indicated in the graphs and recipes are not the same as the ones imprinted on the machine. You need to think about where to set the dial somewhere in the range of 320° and 400°F in the event that you need to cook at 350° or 390°F.

The bin has a nonstick covering and is sufficiently little to go in the dishwasher without hoarding an excess of room. You can pick the Dash with a polished red, water, white, or dark outside.

Pros

• Small

• Doesn't require preheating

• basket is nonstick and dishwasher safe

Cons

• Controls aren't advanced.

• Cooks only one-half pound of food well

Breville Smart Oven Air

You pay as much as possible for the attractive brushed tempered steel Breville Smart Oven Air, yet you get the best in a class toaster oven, notwithstanding an air fryer. In air fryer mode, it consistently turned out crispy food and chicken pieces that tasted fried. The computerized controls are instinctive to program and incorporate programmed preheat. The Breville likewise has a splendid oven light.

In spite of the fact that it's enormous even by toaster oven norms, it can really supplant your oven. No requirement for unique toaster oven-sized cookware here. What's more, Breville claims it can suit a 14-pound turkey.

I do have one significant bandy with this item. The manual doesn't contain any suggestions for what, how much, or to what extent to cook different foods. This may not be an issue for preparing or roasting, however in case you're new to air browning, and you're alone when you're beginning. Additionally, remember the entirety of the parts requires hand washing.

Pros

• It's an air fryer, toaster, and ledge oven.

• Has advanced controls

• Foods turn out crispy.

Cons

• Large

• Manual isn't useful.

• Parts aren't dishwasher safe.

GoWISE USA 8-in-1 Air Fryer XL

The GoWise 8-in-1 Air Fryer XL 5.9 Qt gets along nicely at air broiling and has some pleasant focal points. Notwithstanding a huge limit, it has computerized controls with eight prearranged settings (henceforth the name) and an alert that you can set to remind you to hurl food during cooking. It doesn't require preheating, and the crate is both nonstick covered and dishwasher safe. With the GoWise, you get a cookbook to give you loads of formula thoughts for air broiling. Notwithstanding high contrast, you can browse red and purple lodging.

Pros

• Doesn't require preheating

• Has computerized controls

• Includes formula book

Cons

• Basket is dubious about expelling.

Krups Fast Fry Deluxe Digital Air Fryer

On account of its barrel shape and tempered steel lodging, the Krups East Fry Deluxe Digital Air Fryer 4.2 L is one of the more tasteful looking air fryers available. It yields good outcomes, giving food crunch and light cooking, yet I question you'd have the option to dupe anybody into accepting their fried chicken supper left a profound fat fryer.

It has computerized controls and programmed programs for fundamentals like fries and chicken just as for progressively unordinary ones like flame broiling and cake. The directions for preheating in the manual are confounding, and during testing, I never heard a preheat blare. In the diagrams, temperatures are surrendered, which don't coordinate with the ones that appeared on the showcase. While the container can go in the dishwasher, its nonstick covering makes cleanup moderately simple on the off chance that you pick hand washing.

Pros

• Digital controls

• Basket is nonstick and dishwasher safe.

Cons

• Requires preheating

• It only gives food light crunch and carmelizing.

Farberware 3.2-Quart Digital Oil-Less Fryer

One of the most sensibly evaluated air fryers you can purchase, the Farberware 3.2-Quart Digital Oil-Less Fryer, does a quite great job of crisping and carmelizing, particularly with regards to solidified foods. You do need to make certain to preheat and flip foods over to get even outcomes. As the manual didn't clarify the utilization as plainly as it could have, there was a smidgen of an expectation to absorb information to find a workable pace. At the point when it's a great opportunity to haul the crate out, it sticks a bit. Be that as it may, if the value is your primary concern, you can't beat the Farberware, and it even accompanies an air fryer cookbook. It comes in the dark and white.

Pros

• Reasonably valued

• Includes a Cookbook

• Basket is nonstick and dishwasher safe.

Cons

• Requires preheating

• Basket is dubious about evacuating.

Dark and Decker Crisp 'N Bake Air Fry Toaster Oven

If you just don't have space on your ledge for one more apparatus yet need to bounce broadcasting live fryer pattern, this multitasker may work. Presently, I won't lie, it is anything but an extravagant schmancy ledge oven like the Cuisinart Airfryer Toaster Oven or the Breville Smart Oven Air, the two of which look awesome and can practically trade your oven for everything except for roasting a colossal turkey. Yet, the Black and Decker won't set you back a group. Truth be told, it's more affordable than most air fryers. What's more, notwithstanding air broiling, it does an extremely pleasant activity of making toast and can even prepare a decent cake.

It accompanies a wide bushel, so you can spread out the food which advances cooking, crisping, and makes it simpler to flip foods over for all the more even outcomes. I got the best "broiling" with solidified foods; natively constructed French fries couldn't generally get by, yet battered chicken bosoms turned out beautiful darn great.

The bushel slides in on side backings like the oven rack, yet there's no dish below it or more the heating curls. Notwithstanding hand scouring the tempered steel work container, I needed to wipe consumed on hitter trickles off of the curls. The Black and Decker has a removable dishwasher safe scrap plate. As there's very little information on-air singing in the manual, be set up to research and explore different avenues regarding times and temperatures, just as systems.

Pros

• Reasonably evaluated

• Doesn't require preheating

Cons

• Difficult to clean

• Manual isn't useful.

• Controls aren't computerized

Krups Fry Delight

While the Krups Fry Delight won't give you very as crunchy results as the best air fryers, it likewise won't void your ledger. Before the latest round of testing, it was my best worth pick. I love its square plan, which looks increasingly alluring, as well as makes it simple to bury. While this is one of the littler models, it can even now hold as much as a pound and a portion of fries, 4 chicken pieces, or a pound of meat. It doesn't have computerized controls, and you need to fiddle a piece to set the cooking temp and time effectively. As the network at the base of the bushel isn't nonstick covered, it takes a touch of real effort to get it clean. Yet, for the cash and the size, the Krups is a decent decision. Select either a dark or white lodging.

Pros

• Reasonably estimated

• Holds a ton of food for its size

• Easy to store

Cons

• No computerized controls

• Difficult to clean

Force Air Fryer XL

If that it's somewhat littler in size and limit than many air fryers, the Power Air Fryer XL can cook and fresh around one pound of food without a moment's delay. It has advanced controls with cooking preset projects. I discovered it to some degree, conventional in appearance, and the crate doesn't coast out as easily as on a few. On the positive side, it tidies up in the dishwasher, accompanies a formula booklet, and won't set you back a group.

Pros

• Digital controls

• Holds a ton of food for its size

• Basket is nonstick and dishwasher safe.

Cons

• Basket sticks when it's evacuated.

Dark and Decker 2L Purifry

The egg-formed Black and Decker 2L Purifry isn't too a lot littler in size than other air fryers yet has a lot littler bin. Dark and Decker just suggest that you cook a half-pound of fries or each burger in turn. While it gives great outcomes, it appears as though in case you're devoting such a lot of counter space to an apparatus, you ought to have the option to cook enough food for four on the double. Also, the crate didn't skim in and out effectively. In the same way as others, it doesn't have advanced controls, so it's difficult to set correctly. Be that as it may, my greatest objection is that the numbers are little to such an extent that I truly expected to utilize an amplifying glass to set the temperature. Completions are accessible in highly contrasting.

Pros

• Reasonably evaluated

• Foods turn out crispy.

Cons

• No computerized controls

• Doesn't hold a great deal of food for its size

• Difficult to understand settings

Moment Vortex Plus Air Fryer

This is a case of an item that is genuinely impaired by its manual. Except if you, as of now, have involvement in air browning, we'd suggest you keep away from the Instant Vortex Plus Air Fryer Oven, the principal air fryer from Instant Pot. The "Beginning Guide" accompanies not many proposals with respect to what to cook and no suggestions concerning the amount to cook. Both a bushel and plate are incorporated. While generally, the maker recommends air broiling in the crate, we showed signs of improvement sautéing and crisping when we utilized a plate.

On the advanced control cushion, you'll discover five different capacities, and for them, as well, you're left in obscurity concerning what and the amount to cook and for to what extent. The most one of a kind component is a rotisserie. However, there's very an expectation to learn and adapt for making sense of how to embed the spit and get a chicken pivoting in the oven. In the event that you are happy to place in some experimentation, you will be happy with the Vortex Plus' cooking results. On the in addition to side, there's a brilliant inside light, and the parts are dishwasher safe.

Pros

• Includes a rotisserie

• Bright inside light

• Good cooking results

Cons

• Manual not accommodating

• Confusing to utilize

NuWave Brio Digital Air Fryer 6 Quart

The NuWave Brio Digital Air Fryer 6 Quart is on the huge size and has a major limit. In our tests, it cooked all the more unevenly and gave less searing and crisping than others. Because of computerized controls that are anything but difficult to peruse and program, I found it especially helpful to utilize. It has worked in preheat setting and prearranged settings for things like fries and chunks that you're probably going to cook. A divider for the crate is incorporated with the goal that you can air fry two foods immediately and shield them from blending. In the manual, there's a large number of recipes to assist you with getting great use out of your air fryer. While the parts are dishwasher sheltered, top rack just is suggested, and the container might be unreasonably enormous for the upper rack.

Pros

• Holds a great deal of food

• Has advanced controls

Cons

• Large

• Foods don't turn out crispy.

NuWave Bravo Smart Oven

The NuWave Bravo Smart Oven is a delightful machine with heaps of decent highlights, including two oven racks, a temperature test, and projects for toasting, preparing, and roasting just as air broiling.

Tragically, it truly missed the mark when it came to air searing. Much subsequent to cooking twice the length in each other air fryer, potato strips looked somewhat like French fries. Naturally, breaded chicken pieces turned out pale and spongy. While solidified fries and chunks crisped up fairly, they took far longer than the occasions determined on the bundles. This may be a decent purchase for a toaster oven. However, I don't prescribe it in case you're searching for an air fryer.

Pros

• An air fryer, toaster oven and ledge oven in one

Cons

• Manual not accommodating for air searing

• Food didn't turn out crispy.

• Very long cooking occasions

Oster DuraCeramic Air Fryer

In contrast to most, the Oster DuraCeramic Air Fryer is round and has a transparent top so you can perceive what's going on. It has a separable handle that you cut on to the bowl to expel it after air browning, yet I thought that it was dubious to utilize. For cooking things like fries, there's an instrument to utilize the fryer in a tilted situation to wipe out the need to shake or hurl during cooking. In our cook-off, the Oster took the longest to cook and gave the least crispy aftereffects of everything tried.

Distinction Between Air Fryer And Convection Oven

There's a distinction between an air fryer and a convection oven.

From the start sight, they appear to do a similar activity. The airflow gives the food the required measure of heat for cooking.

The sight-seeing circulation guideline expects practically no oil for food planning.

There are sure contrasts that can assist you with deciding. These subtleties can decide your choices with regards to your new kitchen supply.

Convection Oven versus Air Fryer: Features

Convection ovens and air fryers share a ton of similitudes. The previously mentioned sight-seeing circulation is one of the most significant attributes when looking at these gadgets. We'll attempt to look past those similitudes when contrasting them. Subsequently, you'll get a separation of the main highlights of both convection ovens and air fryers. Along these lines, you'll have the option to figure out which one is all the more engaging for your situation.

In contrast to normal traditional ovens, the best convection ovens, for example, Breville BOV800XL, convey the sight-seeing evenly. Convection ovens, for example, modify the temperature naturally once you place the food in them. This element allows you to try different things with an assortment of dishes.

Convection ovens are typically huge and appropriate for large courses. They offer enough space for a scope of various culinary encounters. With convection ovens, you don't need to stress over your food winding up undercooked. The air dissemination arrives at the center of the food, much the same as it forms the edges.

The best air fryers, among which we essentially should specify Phillips air fryer, represent a culinary development. While you'll most likely utilize a specific measure of oil when cooking with a convection oven, here it isn't vital. Most air fryers have a container where you place the food you need to cook. Despite the fact that they arrive at the pinnacle of their exhibition in singing, you can attempt different strategies with a significant number of them.

The most significant component of air fryers, for example, Power XL air fryer, is that you can put them on your kitchen counter. They are sufficiently minimized to remain on the counter without occupying an excess of room. In the clash of convection ovens versus air fryers, it's essential to call attention to the temperature. As a rule, air fryers arrive at higher temperatures, and are in this way, progressively helpful for sensitive suppers, for example, treats. Convection ovens will, in general, be somewhat excessively hard on this sort of dish.

When examining air fryers versus convection ovens, we could state that air fryers are increasingly helpful on account of the ledge arrangement. In any case, remember that there are convection ovens, for example, convection toaster oven, which is a ledge, also.

Convection Ovens versus Air Fryers: Healthiness

The path both of these gadgets treat the food is amazingly healthy. Convection ovens and air fryers take part in a comparative strategy, which includes sight-seeing circulation. Most of the two classes use fans which deliver and empower the tourist flow all through the unit.

It's critical to bring up the way that, in contrast to regular ovens, these gadgets don't have heating components. The presence of heating components confines the temperature to the zone, which is the closest.

Since this is a relative convection oven versus air fryer survey, we should see which one leads the pack with regards to healthiness.

Enter your Convection ovens do offer various conceivable outcomes. You can cook anything you might envision in these ovens. In contrast to broiling skillet or profound fryers, you can include a modest quantity of oil to your dish. The food will cook in its regular juices, with no compelling reason to include abundance oil. Thusly you can get the characteristic sauce in case you're handling meat.

Then again, the healthier decision on account of convection ovens versus air fryers could be the air fryers.

Upon al, a large portion of the air fryers requires no expansion of oil by any stretch of the imagination. The prefix oil-less stands nearby many air fryers. When preparing or searing in a convection oven, you'll likely add some oil to include some dampness.

Air fryers arrive at higher temperatures. Along these lines, the cooking procedure with them is shorter. Along these lines, your food doesn't dry, and it finds a workable pace healthy fixings. If you utilize the oven to slow-cook, a lot of supplements can evaporate simultaneously.

In any case, cooking with less to no oil is an incredible option for some cooking systems out there.

Convection Ovens versus Air Fryers: Size and Cooking Capacity

These two factors enormously impact the decision of any purchaser, paying little heed to some other components. The quantity of the unit matters since you should adjust it to your kitchen space. There's nothing more awful than having kitchen supplies, which limit your development in the kitchen. This sort of pickle can likewise be hazardous, and it can cause breaking and harming.

To the extent the cooking limit goes, this is a totally abstract issue. You know about your cooking capacities and requirements. Regarding those elements, pick the comparing cooking limit.

Presently, how about we see what to convection ovens and air fryers bring to the table in these particular angles.

Convection ovens are generally greater than air fryers.

Their arrangement is normally not ledge, so a few people discover them not as agreeable as the air fryers. Likewise, you need to curve to put the food into it, to screen the cooking procedure, lastly, to take the food out. This sort of situating might be awkward for you. Air fryers are littler and increasingly smaller in size. In this manner, they fit on kitchen counters, and you can move toward them effectively. They are simpler to store and clean, which we will talk about later.

The greater the size – the greater the cooking limit. For the most part, you'll see that this standard applies to kitchen supplies. Justifiably, convection ovens and air fryers are the same. Since convection ovens are greater, their cooking limit is typically bigger. This implies it'll allow you to cook more food without a moment's delay. Also, you'll have the option to put greater pieces of food in it without slashing it.

Then again, because of their shape, air fryers, for the most part, have a littler cooking limit. Don't let this dolt you. Many air fryers have profound chambers in which you can put a lot of food, for example, French fries. In any case, you won't have the option to roast sheep legs or greater pieces like such.

Convection Ovens versus Air Fryers: Maintenance and Reliability

• No one needs to go through an excess of cash or cash, keeping up their culinary gadgets. Food dribbling, oil splatter, and steady stains can cause a wreck in your kitchen. In case you're not an enthusiast of cleaning, you'll welcome an air fryer much in excess of a convection oven. Many air fryers, for example, T-fal FZ7002 Actifry low-fat multi-cooker, are amazingly simple to clean.

This air fryer specifically has a non-stick container, which will take you just several minutes to clean off. Their inside, just as outside, contains material that doesn't raise any ruckus during cleaning. Likewise, air fryers are littler, and you'll certainly invest less energy looking after it. Its versatility is likewise useful.

With regards to support, convection ovens do will, in general reason some cerebral pain. Convection oven proprietors should focus on and truly get in there. Their situation additionally makes it difficult to arrive at each and every region of the unit. The developed stains and trickling can be very difficult to dispose of. If there should be an occurrence of convection oven cleaning, you'll most likely need to utilize solid cleansers so as to leave it totally perfect.

• Reliability is a relative subject that is difficult to characterize. In this way, it is mistaken to state that both of these classes gives greater unwavering quality. What decides are the materials, the nature of the unit, the settings, and a couple of different parts.

Along these lines, to make certain of dependability, you should respect it for every gadget independently. Give close a to the nature of the structure and the life span of the material. Likewise, the guarantee assumes a noteworthy job in this perspective. A decent guarantee will give you a feeling that all is well with the world, paying little mind to different variables.

On the off chance that we were to by and large talk about unwavering quality, maybe the normally treated steel plan of convection ovens is increasingly alluring.

It is difficult to decide the victor of this convection oven versus air fryer fight. As should be obvious, there are numerous likenesses, and you can draw an equal between these two classes. Likewise, we focused on a portion of the unmistakable highlights of every one of the gadgets.

You can settle on your choice by picking the gadget which contains the most noteworthy number of your preferred qualities.

Despite your choice, it's essential to call attention to that you can't turn out badly with both of these. Consider your desires and your potential outcomes, and "flip the coin."

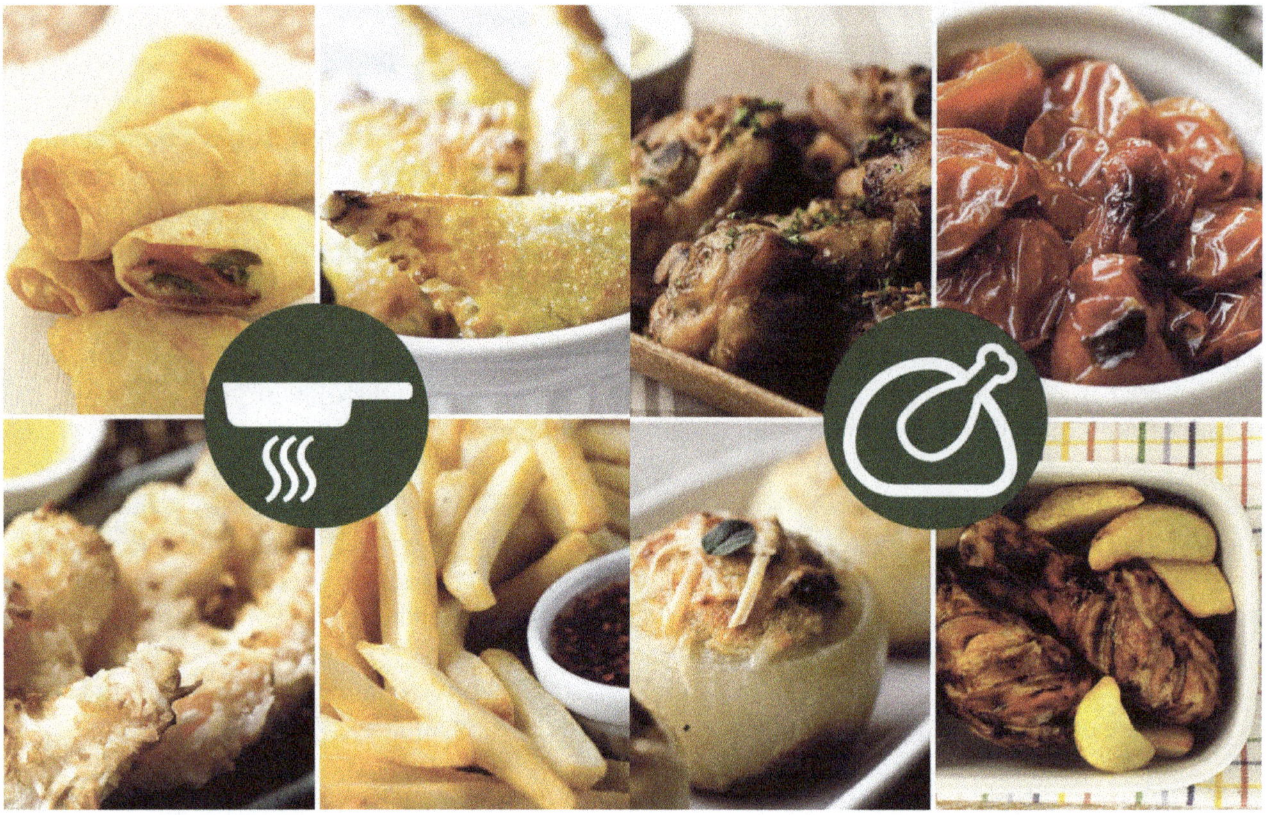

RECIPES

Heavenly Power Air Fryer Oven Recipes

Force Air Fryer Chicken Wings Recipe

The force air fryer can make café quality chicken wings that are delicate, succulent, and delightful. It can bring about extra crispy wings with no fat and included calories. Amass the following fixings and follow my guidelines below to cook your chicken wings utilizing power air fryer oven at home.

Fixings:

- t3 lbs chicken wing pieces cut into drumettes and pads
- Olive oil cooking shower
- 2 tbsp liquefied spread
- 1 tbsp prepared salt
- ½ cup flour
- 3 tbsp maple syrup
- 3 tbsp hot sauce

Guidelines:

Expel tips from chicken wings and separate pads and drumettes. Shower olive oil to gently cover within your air fry container. Spot wings in a medium-size bowl and shower them gently with olive oil splash.

From that point forward, blend the salt and the flour in a medium-size bowl and hurl the wings in the flour blend to be gently covered. Spot your wings in the fryer bushel and afterward into the force air fryer oven. Press the M to fasten and alter the cooking time to 25 minutes at 325 degrees Fahrenheit.

Regulate the temperature to 400 degrees once the wings have gotten marginally dark-colored. While the wings are cooking, blend the softened margarine, maple syrup, and hot sauce.

Take off the wings from the oven when they are crispy and cooked through. Hurl the completely cooked wings with the sauce. At long last, serve your chicken wings with blue cheddar dressing if necessary.

Force Air Fryer Chicken Tenders Recipe

You can utilize the air fryer for heating tasty, delicate and crispy chicken tenders to flawlessness. Chicken tenders are one of my preferred foods since I can whip them together in a matter of moments. Below are my fixings and stunts for making the most delightful chicken tenders without all the chaos.

Fixings:

• 6 chicken tenders, crude

• 3 enormous eggs

• ½ cup flour, white

• 1 cup panko breadcrumbs

• 1 tsp ocean salt

• ½ tsp dark pepper

• 1 tsp olive oil

• ½ cup milk

Guidelines:

In a medium-size bowl, join panko breadcrumbs with olive oil and blend the eggs in with milk in a different bowl. Empty flour into a pot or dish and plunge chicken tenders into the flour first, at that point into the egg blend, lastly into the panko breadcrumbs blend. Preheat the air fryer by setting it to 400 degrees Fahrenheit for around 5 minutes.

Put the breaded tenders into the fry container and spot the fry bushel into the force air fryer XL. Press the M catch and look to the French fries symbol. Press the force catch to begin and modify the cooking time to 14 minutes at 400 degrees Fahrenheit.

Flip the tenders over the following 7 minutes of cooking to dark-colored the opposite side. Evacuate the tenders when the juices run clear, and the pink substance has vanished. You would now be able to serve your completely cooked tenders with your preferred sauce.

Force Air Fryer Oven Bacon Recipe

My Mom and I utilize a ton of bacon in our low carb recipes, and we lean toward utilizing ithe air fryer to make sweet crispy bacon. Bacon is the staple for breakfast, lunch, and supper. In the event that you are a bacon sweetheart, I will tell you the best way to utilize the air fryer for cooking delicious bacon effectively and in a matter of moments.

Fixings:

- Bacon (as much as you want)

Guidelines:

onPreheat your air fryer to 200 degrees Celsius or 390 degrees Fahrenheit. Spot bacon on a solitary layer inside the air fryer container (no issue if some of the overlay or cover). Alter the air fryer to 350 degrees Fahrenheit and cook for around 10 minutes.

Partially through cooking, flip the bacon and keep cooking for an extra 7 minutes until the bacon turns fresh. Move your completely cooked bacon into a plate that is fixed with paper towels to deplete the overabundance oil. Serve your bacon while still hot.

Force Air Fryer Oven Steak Recipe

Cooking steak in an air fryer is entirely clear. This smaller than expected convection oven cooks food by coursing tourists around to accomplish scrumptious and healthy steaks with less oil. Let me tell you the best way to make lean, delicate, and tasty steak the correct way.

Fixings:

- Ribeye steak or New York strip steak
- Kosher salt to taste
- Butter
- Paprika
- Black pepper to taste
- Garlic powder to taste

Guidelines:

Carry the steak to room temperature so it can cook equally. Splash olive oil on all sides of the steak and season with dark pepper,and garlic powder, fit salt, and paprika, .

Drop the steak inside the air fryer crate and cook for 12 minutes. Flip the steak part of the way through cooking to guarantee all sides are equitably cooked. Top your steak with spread and serve right away.

Force Air Fryer French Fries Recipe

An air fryer can make tasty, crispy, and crunchy French fries that look like your preferred eatery quality French fries. On my absolute first endeavor, I made crispy French fries in under 20 minutes. I'm demonstrating how to cause a healthier French fry so you can to feel great about serving your entire family.

Fixings:

- 2-3 Yukon gold potatoes, cleaned
- 1 tbsp extra-virgin olive oil
- Salt and pepper to taste
- Paprika, garlic powder and different seasonings you may like

Guidelines:

Preheat the air fryer by setting it to 360 degrees Fahrenheit. Slash the potatoes to frame French fry states of around 0.5 inches thick. Spot the crude potato cuts in a bowl containing warm water for 10 minutes.

Channel the potato cuts and move them into an enormous bowl. Shower the crude potato cuts in a bowl with olive oil and season liberally with salt, pepper, and your preferred seasonings like bean stew powder, paprika, or garlic powder. Hurl appropriately to cover the potato cuts.

Have your prepared potato cuts masterminded in a solitary layer reporting in real-time fryer container. Cook them for 15 minutes keeping up the temperature of 360 degrees Fahrenheit. When the clock has slipped by, expel the fresh fries from the air fryer utilizing a spatula and serve quickly nearby your most loved plunging sauce.

Force Air Fryer Fried Chicken Recipe

It is anything but difficult to make crispy and heavenly fried chicken in an air fryer. Custom made fried chicken can be flawlessly delicious within and crunchy outwardly – with no additional fat and unhealthy calories. With the following fixings and cooking guide, it won't take well before that amazing smell begins filling the kitchen.

Fixings:

• 4 bits of chicken legs, thighs, or bosoms

• 1 piece egg

• 1 cup universally handy flour

• 1 tsp flavoring salt

• 2 tbsp old straight Cajun flavoring

Directions:
Preheat the air fryer to around 380 degrees F. In a huge bowl, blend 2 tsp old cove flavoring, 1 tsp flavoring salt, and 1 cup generally useful flour. Make a point to whisk the fixings altogether together.

Beat the egg in a different bowl. At that point, dig the chicken pieces in three stages: first, drop the pieces into the flour blend and set them back into the plate: next, dig the chicken pieces in the egg; lastly, drop the pieces again into the flour and shake off the overabundance flour.

Splash the chicken pieces with the oil, guaranteeing each piece gets secured totally. Put the chicken pieces into the base of the fryer container and postion the air fryer to 180 degrees F. and cook for 25 minutes. A moment meat thermometer can assist you with knowing whether it has arrived at 180 degrees Fahrenheit.

Expel the fried chicken from the air fryer. Be cautious while taking out the fried chicken from the air fryer since it very well may be hot. Serve quickly while still hot and appreciate.

Force Air Fryer Grilled Cheese Recipe

You can cook an ideal flame broiled cheddar utilizing an air fryer. Flame-broiled cheddar sandwiches are my go-to snappy supper when I don't have anything arranged. Appreciate a gooey, rich feast with the following fixings and thoughts.

Fixings:

• 2 bread cuts

• 50 g spread or margarine

• 100 g cheddar

• 2 cuts tomato

• 1 cut ham

Guidelines:
Heat the air fryer to 360 degrees Fahrenheit or 180 degrees Celsius, which could take around 3 minutes relying upon the air fryer model you are utilizing. Apply margarine on one side of each bread cut. Ensure you utilize enough spread to get them secured totally.

Cut the cheddar and put it between the two bread cuts. Guarantee the buttered sides are confronting the outside of the sandwich. Put the sandwich in the air fryer crate and cook for 8 minutes.

Inside the initial 4 minutes of cooking, open the crate and flip the flame-broiled cheddar over. At long last, cook for the staying 4 minutes. Evacuate the flame-broiled cheddar when cooked and let it cool before you can appreciate it.
Force Air Fryer Hamburgers Recipe

A succulent air fryer burger works out positively for French fries cooked in the air fryer. A snappy and simple air fryer burger is a hamburger formula that is cherished by numerous individuals, and your entire family will unquestionably adore it. Follow my manual to make delectable and without gluten burgers in an air fryer.

Fixings:

• Ground hamburger

• Salt

• Pepper

• Cheese

• Buns

Guidelines:

Preheat the air fryer to 180 degrees Celsius or 350 degrees Fahrenheit. Join the meat, dark pepper, and salt in a bowl and organize the hamburger blend to shape four burger patties. Shower the bin of the air fryer with a little oil to softly cover.

Include the burgers into the air fryer container. Let it cook for 8-12 minutes relying upon your favored degree of doneness. Flip them over part of the way through cooking to guarantee they are uniformly cooked.

One moment before they are completely cooked, take out the air fryer bin and top every burger with cheddar. Put the air fryer container back and cook until done. At long last, form your burgers and serve to appreciate.

Last Verdict:

Force air fryer ovens are your pass to healthier fried foods which taste crispy, crunchy, and scrumptious. What we have quite recently secured above is our definitive assortment of the best air fryer recipes you can without much of a stretch make at home. Remember that force air fryer oven recipes don't stop at what we have shrouded in our formula aggregation.

You can, too, discover several most loved air fryer recipes for your tidbits, pastries, snacks, the breakfast, lunch, the supper, and the sky is the limit from there. An air fryer really remains your go-to kitchen apparatus on the off chance that you need to appreciate righteous solace foods like chicken wings, fries, onion rings, thus significantly more. You can never lament having an air fryer oven is one of your kitchen munititions stockpiles.

Crispy Buffalo Air Fryer Chicken Wings Recipe

We are almost certain on the off chance that your server these to your loved ones, they will never acknowledge they were not made in a profound fryer!

Fixings:

- 1 lb. chicken wings (new or solidified)

- 1/2 cup Frank's Hot Sauce

- Fat-Free Blue Cheese (discretionary)

Bearings:

1. Preheat air fryer for 3-5 minutes at 380°.

2. Spot chicken wings in a solitary layer in the air fryer.

3. Air fry for 12 minutes at 380°.

4. Flip wings over with tongs and air fry for an additional 12 minutes.

5. You can include your sauce now in the event that you might want – simply include your sauce and mix well with the chicken (I picked to include my sauce in the wake of cooking the wings to keep my air fryer clean – others like to add it during to get the firmness of the flavors on the skin!)

5. R the temperature to 400 degrees and cook for around 5 additional minutes.

6. In the event that you didn't include the sauce during cooking – place the wings in a bowl and include your sauce and hurl or shake until every one of the wings is secured.

7. Present with celery and blue cheddar (discretionary).

The formula, as demonstrated, makes (4) – 4 oz. Servings. By expanding the temperature throughout a previous couple of moments of cooking, you are helping the wings get that smidgen of extra crispy goodness that everybody cherishes!

Weight Watchers data

The air fryer will limit the fat and calories from standard chicken wings – the below are gauges for Smart Points dependent on the Weight Watchers application.

• 4 ounces of chicken (a gauge of 5 chicken wings) with no skin is 4 Smart Points

• 4 ounces of chicken (the gauge of 5 chicken wings) with skin is 8 Smart Points

Guidelines

1. Preheat air fryer for 3-5 minutes at 380°.

2. Place chicken wings in a solitary layer in the air fryer.

3. Air fry for 12 minutes at 380°.

4. Flip wings and air fry for an additional 12 minutes.

5. You can include your sauce now, or toward the finish of your cooking.

6. After the 12 minutes is done - turn the temperature up to 400° and cook for 5 additional minutes

7. Be sure the interior temperature of the wings are 165° before expelling

8. If you didn't include your sauce during the cooking, at that point, place in a bowl and include your favored sauce and shake or hurl until wings are secured.

Notes

Present with celery and blue cheddar (discretionary) and attempt different sauces for various flavors and zest levels.

Chicken Tenders/Fingers Recipe Serves 4

Fixings:

- 1½ lb. of Chicken Tenderloins
- Salt and pepper to taste
- 1 Egg
- 2 tablespoon of Milk
- 1 cup of universally handy Flour
- 1 teaspoon + 1 teaspoon of Garlic Powder
- 1 teaspoon + 1 teaspoon of Paprika
- 1 cup of Panko Breadcrumbs
- GoWise XL Air Fryer
-

Guidelines:

- yLightly season the chicken tenders with salt and pepper.
- Crack the egg in a bowl. Include the milk, salt, and pepper and whisk it well.
- In a shallow bowl, join the flour, salt, and pepper, 1 teaspoon of garlic powder, and 1 teaspoon of paprika. Blend it well.
- In another shallow bowl, join the panko breadcrumbs, salt, and pepper, 1 teaspoon of garlic powder, and 1 teaspoon of paprika. Blend it well.
- Take a chicken delicate. Dig it in the universally handy flour blend. Shake off the abundance. Plunge it in the egg blend. And afterward, cover it totally with the panko breadcrumb blend. Keep it aside on a wire rack.
- Repeat with all the chicken tenders.
- Place scarcely any cuts in the softly lubed air fryer crate, in a solitary layer. Gently splash the piece covered tenders.
- Air fry at 380 F for 14 minutes, flipping at the midway imprint (at 7 minutes).

• Repeat with all the readied chicken tenders.

• Serve your chicken tenders hot with ketchup or farm, or whatever sauce you appreciate them with the most. In our home, we happen to adore a decent nectar mustard dressing.

Air Fryer Chicken Tenders

planning time: 10 MINUTES

cook time: 15 MINUTES

all-out time: 25 MINUTES

Not any more fried chicken fingers for the children with this air fryer form that is similarly as clammy and crispy as the less healthy choice!

Fixings

• 1½ lb. of Chicken Tenderloins

• Salt and pepper to taste

• 1 Egg

• 2 tablespoon of Milk

• 1 cup of universally handy Flour

• 1 teaspoon + 1 teaspoon of Garlic Powder

• 1 teaspoon + 1 teaspoon of Paprika

• 1 cup of Panko Breadcrumbs

Directions

1. hLightly season the chicken tenders with salt and pepper.

2. Crack the egg in a bowl. Include the milk, salt, and pepper and whisk it well.

3. In a shallow bowl, consolidate the flour, salt, and pepper, 1 teaspoon of garlic powder, and 1 teaspoon of paprika. Blend it well.

4. In another shallow bowl, consolidate the panko breadcrumbs, salt, and pepper, 1 teaspoon of garlic powder, and 1 teaspoon of paprika. Blend it well.

5. Take a chicken delicate. Dig it in the generally useful flour blend. Shake off the overabundance. Dunk it in the egg blend. And afterward, cover it totally with the panko breadcrumb blend. Keep it aside on a wire rack.

6. Repeat with all the chicken tenders.

7. Place hardly any cuts in the gently lubed air fryer bushel, in a solitary layer. Gently shower the morsel covered tenders.

8. Air fry at 380 F for 14 minutes, flipping at the midway imprint (at 7 minutes).

9. Repeat with all the readied chicken tenders.

10. Serve hot with ketchup or farm.

Notes

Weight Watchers Freestyle focuses = 6 and shrewd focuses = 9.

Herbed Air Fryer Potato Wedges

yield: 8

planning time: 25 MINUTES

cook time: 15 MINUTES

complete time: 40 MINUTES

Fixings

- 4 huge Russet Potatoes
- 2 teaspoons of minced new Rosemary
- 2 teaspoons of minced new Thyme
- 2 tablespoon of Extra Virgin Olive Oil
- Salt and pepper to taste

Directions

1. Wash and thoroughly scour the potatoes.

2. Slice the potatoes, longwise, down the middle. At that point, cut every half into 2 or 3 wedges, contingent upon the size of the potato.

3. Soak the potato wedges in chilly water for 20 minutes.

4. Drain the legumes potatoes and pat dry the kitchen towel.

5. In an enormous bowl, blend the oil, crisp herbs, salt, and pepper. Blend it well.

6. Toss in the potato wedges. Blend well, ensuring each wedge is totally covered with the oil-herb blend.

7. Lightly oil the air fryer bin with oil fog.

8. Place the potato wedges in a solitary layer. You should cook the potatoes in bunches

9. Air Fry the potato at 350 degrees for 15 minutes, shaking and flipping the wedges after each 5 to 6 minutes.

10. These potato recipe wedges are done in less than 15 to 17 minutes. If you need considerably crispier, air fry for an extra 3 minutes at 400 F.

Notes

• Soaking the potato wedges disposes of the overabundance starch, bringing about crisper fries.

• In a spot of crisp herb, don't hesitate to utilize the dried assortment. You will require just ½ teaspoon of every herb in the dried assortment.

• Smart Points determined with the Weight Watcher's formula manufacturer.

Weight Watchers Donuts

Delightful doughnuts with just 3 SP a piece!

• 1 cup nonfat Greek yogurt

• 1 cup self-rising flour, partitioned

• 1 tablespoon vanilla bean glue

• 1/2 cup cinnamon Splenda blend

• optional: coat (powdered sugar + water blended)

Join nonfat Greek yogurt in addition to 3/4 self-rising flour and 1 tablespoon vanilla bean glue.

Turn out onto a floured surface utilizing the other 1/4 cup flour.

Gap into 5 sections. Move up to make doughnuts.

e Cook in the air fryer at 375* for 4 minutes. Flip over and cook for another 3-4 minutes. (Because of contrasts in elevation, brands of flour, and so on, you may need to cook at 400 for as long as 15 minutes. Remember that if yours are sticky inside.)

Shower with a non-stick cooking splash, at that point dunk in cinnamon and Splenda.

Discretionary: sprinkle with a coat

Simple Air Fryer Steak

Planning Time

10 mins

Cook Time

12 mins

Resting Time

5 mins

Complete Time

27 mins

This simple air fryer steak formula is tasty and heavenly. It is a simple method to cook steak when you can't flame broil out.

Course: Main Course

Cooking: American

Catchphrase: air fryer, fundamental course, steak

Servings: 4 individuals

Calories: 269 kcal

Creator: Jamie

Fixings

- 2 Rib-eye Steak 8 ounces each
- 1 teaspoon Garlic Powder
- Salt and Pepper to taste
- 1 tablespoon Olive Oil

Directions

1. Drizzle a teaspoon of olive oil on one side of both the steak. Focus on it. Flip and shower a teaspoon of oil on the opposite side of both the steaks.

2. Season the two sides of the steaks liberally with salt, crisply split pepper, and garlic powder. Back rub it in.

3. Lightly splash the air fryer container with a non-vaporized olive oil shower.

4. Place the steak in the air fryer crate

5. Air fry at 400 F for 6 minutes Flip the steak and air fry for an additional 6 minutes at 400 F.

6. Let the steak rest for 5 minutes.

7. Slice contrary to what would be expected and serve right away.

Formula Notes

Utilize a moment read thermometer to check the temperature for your steak. We went for Medium (145F)

125F for Rare

135F for Medium Rare

145F for Medium

150F for Medium Well

Weight Watchers focuses: 4 myWW focuses for Purple, Green, and Blue plans. Serving size is 1/2 a steak or 4 ounces.

Air Fryer Cauliflower with Seasonings

Planning Time

10 mins

Cook Time

20 mins

All out Time

30 mins

This Air Fryer Cauliflower with Seasonings is a healthy and scrumptious side dish.

Course: Side Dish

Food: American

Watchword: air fryer, cauliflower, side dish

Servings: 4 individuals

Calories: 58 kcal

Creator: Jamie

Fixings

- 1 enormous head of Cauliflower broken into little florets
- 2 teaspoon of Smoked Paprika
- 1 teaspoon of Garlic Powder
- Salt and Pepper to taste
- Cooking Spray

Guidelines

1. In an enormous bowl, consolidated the washed cauliflower florets, smoked paprika, garlic powder salt, and pepper. Blend well and guarantee every one of the florets is covered with the seasonings.

2. Lightly shower the air fryer bushel with cooking splash.

3. Add the prepared cauliflower florets. Gently splash the highest point of the florets with cooking shower.

4. Air fry at 400 F for 20 minutes, halting and shaking the bin at regular intervals for cooking.

5. Serve hot.

Air Fryer Cauliflower with Seasonings

Sum Per Serving

Calories 58Calories from Fat 9

% Daily Value*

Fat 1g2%

Immersed Fat 1g6%

Sodium 64mg3%

Potassium 660mg19%

Sugars 12g4%

Fiber 5g21%

Sugar 4g4%

Protein 4g8%

Nutrient A 493IU10%

Nutrient C 101mg122%

Calcium 46mg5%

Iron 1mg6%

Air Fryer Popcorn Shrimp

Planning Time

3 mins

Cook Time

10 mins

All out Time

13 mins

It is extremely simple to make Air Fryer Popcorn Shrimp in an air fryer oven. They turn out crispy and delectable.

Course: Appetizer, Main Course

Cooking: American

Catchphrase: air fryer, tidbit, principle course, shrimp

Servings: 7 individuals

Calories: 230 kcal

Creator: Jamie

Fixings

• 20 ounces breaded popcorn shrimp solidified

Guidelines

1. Put the solidified shrimp in an even layer reporting in real-time fryer food plate.

2. Put the plate into the air fryer oven. R the oven on to 350 degrees F and set the clock for 10 minutes.

3. When the oven is finished cooking expel the plate from the oven, and the shrimp are prepared to serve.

SIMPLE AIR FRYER VEGETABLES

The air fryer is extraordinary for such a large number of recipes; however, making veggies is one of my top choices for the air fryer.

Veggie leaves the air fryer practically great, and children appear to prefer them better as such.

It is an incredible method to go through those new vegetables before they ruin.

Elements FOR AIR FRYER GREEN BEANS

This simple green bean formula just has four fixings. Three of these you likely consistently have available, so all you have to go out, and a purchase is the green beans.

- Fresh Green Beans
- Olive Oil Cooking Spray
- Himalayan Pink Sea Salt
- Black Pepper

The most effective method to MAKE AIR FRYER GREEN BEANS

These air fryer green beans are so natural to make you scarcely even need a formula.

Stage ONE: PREPARE GREEN BEANS

Start off by washing the crisp green beans.

Trim the closures off the green beans, with the kitchen shears.

Stage TWO: SEASON GREEN BEANS

Spot the oiled green beans into an enormous bowl and sprinkle with salt and pepper to taste.

Stage THREE: AIR FRY GREEN BEANS

Presently place the green beans in a solitary layer in the bin of the air fryer. Laying them in a solitary line will enable the green beans to be crisper.

Air fry at 400 degrees for around 8 minutes. Give the bushel a shake part of the way through the cooking time.

At the point when the parts of the bargains beans begin to dark-colored, you will realize they are finished cooking.

Air Fryer Lemon Pepper Shrimp

Planning Time

5 mins

Cook Time

10 mins

Complete Time

15 mins

Air Fryer Lemon Pepper Shrimp is healthy and delectable. This is likewise an extraordinary primary dish Weight Watchers formula with low focuses per serving.

Course: Main Course

Cooking: American

Catchphrase: principle course, shrimp, Weight Watchers

Servings: 2 individuals

Calories: 237 kcal

Fixings

• 1/2 tablespoon olive oil

• 1 Lemon squeezed

• 1 tsp lemon pepper

• ¼ tsp paprika

• ¼ tsp garlic powder

• 12 ounces uncooked medium shrimp stripped and deveined

• 1 lemon cut

Directions

1. Join olive oil, lemon juice, lemon pepper, paprika, and garlic powder in a bowl.

3. Include shrimp and throw until secured.

4. Spot shrimp in the air fryer and cook until pink and firm, 6 to 8 minutes. Present with lemon cuts.

5. For additional flavor, you can pour any additional marinade over the shrimp in the air fryer before cooking. This is discretionary.

Formula Notes

Separation of the cooked shrimp into 2 servings, and each serving is 1 Point for Blue and Purple plans and is three focuses for the Green arrangement.

Weight Watchers Air Fryer Apple Chips with Cinnamon

Planning Time

10 mins

Cook Time

10 mins

Resting Time

10 mins

All out Time

20 mins

Air fryer apple chips with cinnamon are an extraordinary nibble for Weight Watchers. This zero-point Weight Watchers formula is crunchy and heavenly, thus simple to make.

Course: Snack

Food: American

Watchword: canapé, apples, healthy, nibble

Servings: 4 individuals

Calories: 51 kcal

Fixings

• 2 apples, any assortment daintily cut, strip left on

• 2 tsp ground Cinnamon stored

Guidelines

1. Cut the apple fifty-fifty and afterward meagerly cut the apple. Try not to utilize the center.

2. Toss the apple cuts with ground cinnamon in a bowl.

3. Spread the apples equitably reporting in real-time fryer container. You may need to do it in bunches, contingent upon the size of your air fryer.

4. Air fry at 350 for 10 minutes, halting and shaking the crate. A portion of the chips will fresh up quicker, contingent upon their thickness. Continue evacuating them occasionally, to abstain from burning. A few cuts may stay together, continue isolating. The apple chip gets crispier while they cool. So if some are still delicate yet look got dried out, separate them, and them with fresh up when cool.

Formula Notes

Since there is no oil utilized in this formula, it is zero Freestyle SmartPoints.

AIR FRYER BEEF EMPANADAS

PREP TIME:10 mins

COOK TIME:16 mins

Absolute TIME:30 mins

YIELD:8 SERVINGS

COURSE: Appetizer, Dinner, Lunch

CUISINE: American

These simple meat empanadas made with my natively constructed hamburger picadillo filling and locally acquired empanada mixture are "fried" in the air fryer for empanadas that territory prepared in minutes (just takes 8 minutes to cook)!

Fixings

• 8 Goya empanada circles, in solidified area, defrosted

• 1 cup picadillo

• 1 egg white, whisked

• 1 teaspoon water

Guidelines

1. Preheat the air fryer to 325F for 8 minutes. Shower the container liberally with cooking splash.

2. Place 2 tbsp of picadillo in the focal point of each circle. Overlap into equal parts and utilize a fork to seal the edges. Rehash with the rest of the mixture.

3. Whisk the egg whites with water, at that point, brush the highest points of the empanadas.

4. Bake 2 or 3 at once in the air fryer 8 minutes, or until brilliant. Expel from heat and rehash with the remaining empanadas.

Serving: 1empanada, Calories: 183kcal, Carbohydrates: 22g, Protein: 11g, Fat: 5g, Saturated Fat: 1g, Cholesterol: 16mg, Sodium: 196mg, Fiber: 1g, Sugar: 2.5g

Blue Smart Points:5

Green Smart Points:5

Purple Smart Points:5

Focuses +:5

Air Fryer Pork Taquitos

yield: 10 SERVINGS

Delightful pork or chicken taquitos that are only 8 Weight Watchers Smart Points.

Fixings

• 3 cups cooked destroyed pork tenderloin or chicken

• 2 1/2 cups fat-free destroyed mozzarella

• 10 little flour tortillas

• 1 lime, squeezed

• Cooking shower

Guidelines

1. Preheat air fryer to 380 degrees.

2. Sprinkle lime squeeze over pork and delicately blend around.

3. Microwave 5 tortillas one after another with a moist paper towel over it for 10 seconds, to relax.

4. Add 5 oz. of pork and 1/4 cup of cheddar to a tortilla.

5. Tightly and delicately move up the tortillas.

6. Line tortillas on a lubed foil-lined skillet.

7. Spray an even layer of cooking shower over tortillas.

8. Air Fry for 8-11 minutes until tortillas are a brilliant shading, flipping partially through.

9. 2 taquitos per serving WW SP - 8.

10. But if you don't have an air fryer, they can likewise be prepared in the oven for 8 - 10 minutes on 375 degrees.

Notes

1. Recommend 2 taquitos per serving

2. Add discretionary things like salsa or harsh cream to plunge!

3. Serve with guacamole and make a light feast that everybody will adore.

4. Weight Watchers Smart Points determined to utilize the Weight Watchers formula developer.

AIR FRYER SWEET POTATO FRIES

PREP TIME:10 mins

COOK TIME:10 mins

All out TIME:20 mins

YIELD:2 SERVINGS

COURSE: Side Dish, Snack

The Crispy sweet potato fries made in the air-fryer, with only a modest quantity of oil! Making them the recipe in the air fryer is such a great amount of healthier than broiling, and decreases the fat and calories, without relinquishing taste.

Fixings

• 2 medium stripped sweet potatoes, 12 oz all out

• 2 teaspoons olive oil

• 1/2 tsp fit salt

• 1/2 teaspoon garlic powder

• 1/4 teaspoon sweet paprika

• fresh dark pepper, to taste

Guidelines

1. Preheat air fryer to 400°F 8 minutes.

2. Lightly shower the fryer bin with oil.

3. Slice every potato into even 1/4 inch thick fries.

4. Toss with oil, salt, garlic powder, dark pepper, and paprika.

5. Cook in 2 or 3 clusters, without congestion the skillet 8 minutes, turning midway.

Serving: 1sweet potato, Calories: 221kcal, Carbohydrates: 42g, Protein: 3g, Fat: 5g, Sodium: 302mg, Fiber: 5g, Sugar: 7g

Blue Smart Points:7

Green Smart Points:7

Purple Smart Points:2

Focuses +:3

AIR FRYER FRENCH FRIES

PREP TIME:5 mins

COOK TIME:15 mins

Complete TIME:20 mins

YIELD:1 SERVING

COURSE: Side Dish, Snack

CUISINE: American

The Crispy french fries made in the air-fryer, with only a limited quantity of oil!

Fixings

- nonstick splash
- 1 medium potato, 6 oz, Yukon gold or reddish-brown, washed and dried
- 1 teaspoon olive oil
- 1/8 teaspoon legitimate salt
- 1/8 teaspoon garlic powder
- fresh broke dark pepper, to taste
- grated Parmesan cheddar, discretionary

Directions

1. Preheat the air fryer 380°F.

2. Cut the potato longwise into 1/4 inch slim cuts; at that point, cut each cut into 1/4 inch fries. (A mandolin is useful here).

3. In a medium bowl, hurl the potatoes and oil. Season with salt, garlic powder, and dark pepper to taste; hurl to cover.

4. Place the potatoes in the container in an even layer without covering or swarming, cook the potatoes 12 to 15 minutes, turning most of the way until fresh.

5. Incase you have a Cuisinart Toaster Style Fryer, cook 350F 12 minutes.

Serving: Potatoes, Calories: 175kcal, Carbo: 32.0g,
Blue Smarter Points:5

Green Smarter Points:5

Purple Smarter Points:1

Focuses +:5

AIR FRYER CHICKEN NUGGETS

All out TIME:20 mins

YIELD: SERVINGS

COURSE: Dinner, Lunch, Snack

CUISINE: American

Making handcrafted Chicken Nuggets in the air-fryer is such a great amount of healthier than cheap food or solidified chunks, thus simple to make.

Fixings

- 16 oz 2 enormous skinless, boneless chicken bosoms, cut into even 1-inch reduced down pieces
- 1/2 teaspoon genuine salt and dark pepper, to taste
- 2 teaspoons olive oil
- 6 tablespoons entire wheat Italian prepared breadcrumbs
- 2 tablespoons panko

• 2 tablespoons ground parmesan cheddar

• olive oil shower, I utilized my Misto

Guidelines

1. Pre-heat the air fryer to 400°F for 8 minutes.

2. Pour the olive oil in one bowl and the breadcrumbs, panko and parmesan cheddar in another.

3. Season the chicken with salt and pepper, at that point, pour iin the bowl with the olive oil and blend it well, so the olive oil equitably covers the entirety of the chicken.

4. Put a couple of lumps of chicken at once into the breadcrumb blend to cover, at that point on the crate.

5. Lightly shower the top with olive oil splash at that point air fry 8 minutes, turning midway. Until brilliant.

CHICKEN PARMESAN IN THE AIR FRYER

PREP TIME:5 mins

COOK TIME:10 mins

Absolute TIME:15 mins

YIELD:4 SERVINGS

COURSE: Dinner

CUISINE: American, Italian

Chicken Parmesan turns out incredible in the Air Fryer, no compelling reason to utilize such a lot of oil!

Fixings

• 2 around 8 oz every chicken bosom, cut down the middle to make 4 more slender cutlets

• 6 tbsp prepared breadcrumbs, and I utilized entire wheat, you can utilize without gluten

• 2 tbsp ground Parmesan cheddar

• 1 tbsp spread, liquefied (or olive oil)

• 6 tbsp decreased fat mozzarella cheddar, and I utilized Polly-o

• 1/2 cup marinara

• cooking splash

Directions

1. Preheat the air fryer 360F° for 3 minutes.

2. Combine breadcrumbs and parmesan cheddar in a bowl. Liquefy the spread in another bowl.

3. Lightly brush the spread onto the chicken, at that point dunk into breadcrumb blend.

4. When the air fryer is prepared, place 2 pieces in the crate and splash the top with oil.

5. Cook 6 minutes, turn and top each with 1 tbsp sauce and 1/2 tbsp of destroyed mozzarella cheddar.

6. Cook 3 additional minutes or until cheddar is dissolved.

7. Set aside and keep warm, rehash with the staying 2 pieces.

Serving: 1piece, Calories: 251kcal, Carbohydrates: 14g, Protein: 31.5g, Fat: 9.5g, Saturated Fat: 3.5g, Cholesterol: 14mg, Sodium: 829mg, Fiber: 1.5g

Blue Smart Points:4

Green Smart Points:7

Purple Smart Points:5

Focuses +:6

AIR FRYER FRENCH FRIES

PREP TIME:5 mins

COOK TIME:15 mins

All out TIME:20 mins

YIELD:1 SERVING

COURSE: Side Dish, Snack

The Crispy french fries made in the air-fryer, with only a modest quantity of oil!

Fixings

- nonstick shower
- 1 medium potato, 6 oz, Yukon gold or reddish-brown, washed and dried
- 1 teaspoon olive oil
- 1/8 teaspoon genuine salt
- 1/8 teaspoon garlic powder
- fresh split dark pepper, to taste
- grated Parmesan cheddar, discretionary

Guidelines

1. Preheat the air fryer 380°F.

2. Cut the potato the long way into 1/4 inch slight cuts; at that point, cut each cut into 1/4 inch fries. (A mandolin is useful here).

3. In a medium bowl, hurl the potatoes and oil. Season with salt, garlic powder, and dark pepper to taste; hurl to cover.

4. Place the potatoes in the crate in an even layer without covering or swarming, cook the potatoes 12 to 15 minutes, turning most of the way until fresh.

Prepared CHICKEN CORDON BLEU

PREP TIME:10 mins

COOK TIME:25 mins

Absolute TIME:35 mins

YIELD:6 SERVINGS

COURSE: Dinner

CUISINE: American

This healthy Chicken Cordon Bleu formula is a family top pick! Loaded down with ham and cheddar at that point breaded and prepared in the oven or made in the air fryer.

Fixings

- cooking shower
- 12 flimsy cut, 36 oz all out skinless, boneless chicken bosoms, 3 oz each
- salt and crisp broke pepper
- 1 enormous egg
- 2 enormous egg whites
- 1 tbsp water
- 1/2 cup prepared breadcrumbs
- 1/4 cup ground parmesan cheddar
- 5 oz 6 cuts meagerly cut lean shop ham, cut into equal parts
- 6 cuts 4.4 oz Sargento diminished fat Swiss cheddar, cut down the middle

Guidelines

1. Preheat oven to 450°F. Shower a huge non-leave heating sheet with a cooking splash.

2. Wash and dry the chicken cutlets; delicately pound the chicken to make more slender and daintily season with salt and dark pepper.

3. Put the chicken on a working surface and spot a cut of ham over the chicken, at that point the cheddar and move, putting them aside crease side down.

4. In 1 medium bowl, whisk eggs and egg whites alongside water to make an egg wash.

5. In another medium bowl, consolidate breadcrumbs and parmesan cheddar.

6. Dip the chicken into the egg wash, at that point, into the breadcrumbs.

7. Place chicken onto the heating sheet appear to be side down. Shower the highest point of the chicken with all the more cooking splash and heat around 25 minutes, or until cooked.

Air Fryer Directions

1. Follow strides over 1 through 6.

2. Preheat the air fryer to 400F. Shower the two sides of the chicken with oil. Cook, in two clusters, 12 minutes turning midway.

Serving: 2pieces, Calories: 378kcal, Carbohydrates: 8g, Protein: 55g, Fat: 10g, Sodium: 813mg, Fiber: 0.5g, Sugar: 1g

Blue Smart Points:3

Green Smart Points:6

Purple Smart Points:3

Focuses +:8

THE CRISPY BREADED PORK CHOPS IN THE AIR FRYER

PREP TIME:10 mins

COOK TIME:12 mins

All out TIME:22 mins

YIELD:6

COURSE: Dinner

CUISINE: American

These Crispy Boneless Breaded Pork Chops turn out wet within and crispy outwardly! P in the air fryer, so they took only 12 minutes to cook.

Fixings

• olive oil shower

• 6 3/4-inch thick focus cut boneless pork slashes, fat cut (5 oz each)

• kosher salt

• 1 enormous egg, beaten

• 1/2 cup panko morsels, checkmarks for GF

• 1/3 cup squashed cornflakes morsels

• 2 tbsp ground parmesan cheddar, discard for dairy-free

• 1 1/4 tsp sweet paprika

• 1/2 tsp garlic powder

• 1/2 tsp onion powder

• 1/4 tsp bean stew powder

• 1/8 tsp dark pepper

Guidelines

1. Prepare and Preheat the air fryer to 400F for 12 minutes and softly shower the bin with oil.

2. Season pork hacks on the two sides with 1/2 tsp genuine salt.

3. Combine panko, cornflake pieces, parmesan cheddar, 3/4 tsp genuine salt, paprika, garlic powder, onion powder, bean stew powder, and dark pepper in a huge shallow bowl.

4. Place the beaten egg in another. Dunk the pork into the egg, at that point scrap blend.

5. When the air fryer is prepared, place 3 of the hacks into the readied container and spritz the top with oil.

6. Cook 12 minutes are turning midway, spritzing the two sides with oil. Put in a safe spot and rehash with the remaining.

Serving: 1pork cleave, Calories: 378kcal, Carbohydrates: 8g, Protein: 33g, Fat: 13g, Cholesterol: 121mg, Sodium: 373mg, Sugar: 1g

Blue Smart Points:7

Green Smart Points:7

Purple Smart Points:7

Focuses +:7

AIR FRYER CHICKEN NUGGETS

Complete TIME:20 mins

YIELD:4 SERVINGS

COURSE: Dinner, Lunch, Snack

CUISINE: American

Making handcrafted Chicken Nuggets in the air-fryer is such a great amount of healthier than inexpensive food or solidified chunks, thus simple to make.

Fixings

- 16 oz 2 enormous skinless, boneless chicken bosoms, cut into even 1-inch scaled-down pieces
- 1/2 teaspoon fit salt and dark pepper, to taste
- 2 teaspoons olive oil
- 6 tablespoons entire wheat Italian prepared breadcrumbs
- 2 tablespoons panko
- 2 tablespoons ground parmesan cheddar
- olive oil shower, I utilized my Misto

Guidelines

1. Pre-heat the air fryer to 400°F for 8 minutes.

2. Pour the olive oil in one bowl and the breadcrumbs, panko and parmesan cheddar in another.

3. Season chicken with salt and pepper, at that point, pour it tin the container with the olive oil and it blend well, so the olive oil equitably covers the entirety of the chicken.

4. Put a couple of pieces of chicken at once into the breadcrumb blend to cover, at that point on the bushel.

5. Lightly splash the top with olive oil shower at that point air fry 8 minutes, turning midway. Until brilliant.

Serving: 4oz chicken, Calories: 188kcal, Carbohydrates: 8g, Protein: 25g, Fat: 4.5g, Saturated Fat: 1g, Cholesterol: 57mg, Sodium: 427mg, Sugar: 0.5g

Blue Smart Points:3

Green Smart Points:5

Purple Smart Points:3

Focuses +:4

ZA'ATAR LAMB CHOPS

PREP TIME:5 mins

COOK TIME:10 mins

Absolute TIME:15 mins

YIELD:4 SERVINGS

COURSE: Dinner

CUISINE: American

Flame-broiled sheep flank slashes prepared with Za'atar, a Mediterranean mix of sumac, thyme, sesame, and salt.

Fixings

- 8 sheep midsection cleaves, cut (about 3.5 oz each bone-in)
- 3 cloves garlic, squashed
- 1 teaspoon extra-virgin olive oil
- 1/2 new lemon
- 1 1/4 teaspoon legitimate salt
- 1 tbsp Za'atar
- fresh ground pepper, to taste

Directions

Flame broil or Broil Method:

1. Rub the sheep hacks with oil and garlic.

2. Squeeze the lemon over the two sides, then season with salt, zatar, and dark pepper.

3. Grill on an outside barbecue or indoor flame broil container over medium-high heat to wanted preferring, for 4 to 5 min. Each side or cook inside the oven on the top rack, 4 to 5 minutes on each side.

Air Fryer Methods:

1. Rub the sheep hacks with oil and garlic.

2. Squeeze the lemon over the two sides, then a season with salt, zatar, and dark pepper.

3. Preheat the air fryer to 400F. In bunches in an even layer, cook to wanted enjoying, around 4 to 5 minutes on each side.

4. My cleaves had 2 1/2 oz crude meat on each bone, and nutritional data is dependent on that.

LEFTOVER TURKEY POT PIE EMPANADAS

PREP TIME:10 mins

COOK TIME:30 mins

Absolute TIME:40 mins

YIELD:10 EMPANADAS

COURSE: Appetizer, Lunch

These remaining Turkey Pot Pie Empanadas or hand pies are a delightful method to go through your extra Thanksgiving turkey!

Fixings

- 1 teaspoon unsalted spread
- 1/4 cup cleaved onion

- 1/4 cup cleaved celery
- 2 tablespoons cleaved crisp parsley

- 1 1/4 cups remaining destroyed cooked turkey bosom, 5 ounces
- 3/4 cup solidified peas and carrots
- 3/4 teaspoon genuine salt
- 1/8 tsp ground dark pepper
- 1/2 tsp dried thyme
- 10 solidified Goya Empanada Discos, the ones for preparing, defrosted
- Cooking splash
- 1 huge egg, whisked

Directions

1. Heat a skillet over medium heat, liquefy margarine. Include onion, celery, and parsley cooking until onions are translucent. Include minced garlic, cooking for an extra moment.

2. Combine the juices and cornstarch together and blend well.

3. Add the turkey, solidified peas and carrots, 3/4 teaspoon salt, pepper, thyme, and juices, mix and cook medium heat, heat to the point of boiling at that point cook until thickened and heated through 2-3 minutes.

4. Place a circle on your work surface. Take 2 tablespoons of the turkey blend and spot in each circle. Utilizing a cake brush, place the egg wash on the external edges of the circle. Overlap the plate over and delicately press the edges to make a seal. Utilize a fork and press around the edges to seal.

5. Brush the egg wash more than one side of each of the empanadas.

6. Spray the preparing sheet with oil, heat 350F 26 to 30 minutes, until brilliant.

Air Fryer:

1. Spray the bushel with oil to forestall staying, move to the crate, in clusters and cook at 380F° for 8 minutes, turning midway. Eat hot.

Focuses +:5

MODEST CHOCOLATE CHIP BANANA BREAD LOAVES

Complete TIME:1 hr

YIELD:12 SERVINGS

COURSE: Breakfast, Brunch, Snack

Entire wheat smaller than usual banana bread made with ready bananas and chocolate chips makes certain to leave a grin all over.

Fixings

- 3 ready medium bananas
- 1/3 cup unsweetened fruit purée
- 1 1/4 cups white entire wheat flour
- 3/4 tsp preparing pop
- 1/4 tsp salt
- 2 tbsp spread, mollified
- 1/3 cup dark colored sugar
- 2 huge egg whites
- 1/2 tsp vanilla concentrate
- 1 1/2 oz small chocolate chips
- Smart Balance preparing shower

Directions

1. Preheat oven to 325°. Splash a non-stick portion skillet with a cooking shower.

2. Mash bananas in a bowl put in a safe spot.

3. In a medium bowl, join flour, heating pop, and salt with a wire whisk. Put in a safe spot.

4. In an enormous bowl cream margarine and sugar with an electric blender.

5. Add egg whites, bananas, fruit purée, vanilla; beat at medium speed until thick. Scratch drawbacks of the bowl.

6. Add flour blend, at that point mix at low speed until joined. Overlap in chocolate chips. Don't over blend.

7. Pour hitter into biscuit skillet; heat on the inside rack for around 40 min.

Serving: 1mini portion, Calories: 198kcal, Carbohydrates: 41g, Protein: 4g, Fat: 5g, Sodium: 222mg, Fiber: 4g, Sugar: 22g

Blue Smart Points:6

Green Smart Points:6

Purple Smart Points:6

Focuses +:6

CHICKEN SAUSAGE BROWN RICE STUFFING WITH CELERY AND MUSHROOMS

Complete TIME:45 mins

YIELD:14 SERVINGS

COURSE: Dinner, Side Dish

Dark-colored rice stuffing made with Italian chicken wiener, celery, mushrooms, and onions. Serve this as a Thanksgiving side dish, or you can even appreciate this as dinner. It's so acceptable and normally gluten-free!

Fixings

- 1 1/2 cups dark colored rice
- 3 1/2 cups water

- 1 chicken bouillon, I utilized Knorr
- 5 joins, 14 oz crude sweet Italian chicken or turkey wiener (I utilized in the open air)
- 2 tbsp olive oil
- 6 celery stalks, hacked
- 1 huge onion, hacked
- 16 oz cut new mushrooms
- salt and new broke pepper to taste

Directions

1. Cook dark colored rice in water and chicken bouillon as per bundle headings.

2. While the rice is cooking, in an enormous substantial saute container, cook chicken wiener on medium heat, separating the meat into little pieces as it cooks until the frankfurter is cooked through and is sautéed. Put aside on a dish.

3. Add olive oil to the container and include the onion, sauté one moment, include the celery, salt, and pepper to taste; cook around 12 minutes, until celery is delicate.

4. Add the mushrooms to the container, progressively salt and pepper if necessary and cook, mixing 5 minutes, at that point cook secured for 2 minutes, or until the mushrooms have discharged their juice and are cooked through.

5. Add the wiener and the cooked rice to the dish and blend well.

NOTES

Calories: 107kcal, Carbohydrates: 16.5g, Protein: 3.5g, Fat: 3g, Sodium: 220mg, Fiber: 1.5g, Sugar: 1g

Blue Smart Points:4

Green Smart Points:4

Purple Smart Points:1

Focuses +:3

CHICKEN AND ZUCCHINI NOODLE CAPRESE

PREP TIME:10 mins

COOK TIME:20 mins

Absolute TIME:30 mins

YIELD:2 SERVINGS

COURSE: Dinner, Lunch

Chicken and Zucchini Noodle Caprese are made with sauteed scaled-down chicken bosom and grape tomatoes cooked with spiralized zucchini, new mozzarella, and basil. A simple, low-carb 30-minute supper!

Fixings

- 1/2 lb boneless skinless chicken bosom, cut 1/2-inch 3D squares
- kosher salt
- 1/4 teaspoon dried oregano
- 1 tablespoon olive oil
- 3 garlic cloves, hacked
- 3/4 lb grape tomatoes, cut down the middle
- pinch squashed red pepper pieces
- Kosher Salt and crisply ground dark pepper, to taste.
- 1 tbsp cleaved new basil
- 1 enormous zucchini, spiralized with Blade D
- 2 oz crisp smaller than normal mozzarella balls, cut down the middle

Guidelines

1. Start by spiralizing the zucchini utilizing cutting edge D in the event that you have the Inspiralizer, or the thickest noodle sharp edge your spiralizer has.

2. Add Season to the chicken with 1/4 teaspoon salt, pepper, and oregano.

3. In an enormous non-stick container set over medications high heat, heat 1/2 tablespoon of the oil.

4. Add the chicken and cook, blending until sautéed and cooked through around 6 minutes. Put in a safe spot.

5. Reduce heat to medium, including the rest of the oil and garlic, and cook until brilliant, 30 seconds. Include the tomatoes, and squashed red pepper pieces, and season with 1/4 teaspoon salt and dark pepper.

6. Reduce the heat to low. Stew, secured, until the tomatoes relax, 15 minutes.

7. Increase heat to high, mix in the zucchini and basil, season with 1/4 teaspoon salt and cook 2 minutes.

8. Add the chicken back to the skillet alongside the mozzarella and serve immediately.

Serving: 2cups, Calories: 342kcal, Carbohydrates: 14g, Protein: 34g, Fat: 17g, Saturated Fat: 5g, Cholesterol: 105mg, Sodium: 808mg, Fiber: 4g, Sugar: 2g

Blue Smart Points:3

Focuses +:9

Flame-broiled PINEAPPLE

YIELD:8 SERVINGS

COURSE: Dessert

Fixings

For the marinade:

- 2 tbsp dull nectar
- 1 tsp olive oil
- 1 tbsp new lime juice
- 1 tsp ground cinnamon
- 8 pineapple cuts, 1/2 inch thick

Directions

1. In a little bowl, consolidate the nectar, olive oil, lime juice, and cinnamon and rush to mix. Put in a safe spot.

2. Heat the flame broil or a barbecue skillet.

3. Lightly coat with cooking splash.

4. Lightly brush the pineapple with the marinade.

5. Grill turning once and treating more than once with the rest of the marinade, until delicate and brilliant, around 3-4 minutes on each side.

6. Serve warm.

Serving: 1slice , Calories: 51kcal, Carbohydrates: 12g, Protein: 0.3g, Fat: 0.8g, Sodium: 0.9mg, Fiber: 0.9g, Sugar: 10.4g

Blue Smart Points:2

Green Smart Points:2

Purple Smart Points:2

Focuses +:1

Hacked FETA SALAD

PREP TIME:15 mins

Complete TIME:15 mins

The hacked serving of mixed greens with romaine lettuce, Feta cheddar, cucumbers, red onion, and dill hurled with a straightforward red wine vinaigrette. A simple side is serving of mixed greens to go with all your Mediterranean dishes.

Fixings

- 8 cups slashed romaine lettuce
- 1/2 English cucumber, stripped and diced in enormous pieces
- 1/3 cup Feta cheddar, disintegrated

- 1/8 little red onion, cut the long way
- 1/4 cup olive oil
- 2 tablespoon red wine vinegar
- 1 1/2 tablespoons crisp hacked dill
- 1/2 teaspoon fit salt
- fresh dark pepper, to taste

Guidelines

1. Toss every fixings together and serve immediately.

Serving: 2cups, Calories: 173kcal, Carbohydrates: 4.5g, Protein: 4g, Fat: 16.5g, Saturated Fat: 3.5g, Cholesterol: 11mg, Sodium: 289mg, Fiber: 2g, Sugar: 2.5g

Blue Smart Points:5

Purple Smart Points:5

Focuses +:5

Herbed Air Fryer Potato Wedges

yield: 8

planning time: 25 MINUTES

cook time: 15 MINUTES

all-out time: 40 MINUTES

Fixings

- 4 enormous Russet Potatoes
- 2 teaspoons of minced new Rosemary
- 2 teaspoons of minced new Thyme
- 2 tablespoon of Extra Virgin Olive Oil
- Salt and pepper to taste

Directions

1. Wash and thoroughly scour the potatoes.

2. Slice the potatoes, longwise, down the middle. At that point, cut every half into 2 or 3 wedges, contingent upon the size of the potato.

3. Soak the potato wedges in chilly water for 20 minutes.

4. Drain all the potatoes and pat dry the kitchen towel.

5. In a huge bowl, blend the oil, new herbs, salt, and pepper. Blend it well.

6. Toss in the potato wedges. Blend well, ensuring each wedge is totally covered with the oil-herb blend.

7. Lightly oil the air fryer crate with oil fog.

8. Place the potato wedges in a solitary layer. You should cook the potatoes in bunches

9. Air-Fry at 350 degrees for 15 min., shaking and flipping the wedges after each 5 to 6 minutes.

10. The potato wedges are completed in 15 to 17 minutes. In the event that you need considerably crispier air fry for an extra 3 minutes at 400 F.

Notes

- Soaking the potato wedges disposes of the overabundance starch, bringing about crisper fries.
- In the spot of crisp herb, don't hesitate to utilize the dried assortment. You will require just ½ teaspoon of every herb in the dried assortment.
- Smart Points determined with the Weight Watcher's formula developer.

AIR FRYER BAKED POTATOES

Air Fryer Baked Potatoes – Make impeccably cooked heated potatoes in the air fryer! You'll never need to utilize your oven again. The skin will be crispy outwardly and consummately delicate and delicate in the center.

Rather than utilizing your oven to make a heated potato, you can utilize an air fryer. Typically, prepared potatoes take in any event an hr relying upon the size of them. Both of these potatoes

that I utilized were around 200 grams for every potato. That is 7 oz. It's simpler to gauge potatoes in grams than ounces on the scale.
Elements FOR AIR FRYER BAKED POTATOES

- 2 Idaho or Russet medium potatoes – I lean toward either Russets or Idado potatoes for this.

- Cooking Spray, for example, Pam – this enables the potato to skin get extra crispy in the event that you like to eat the skin of the potato. I was informed that is the place all the fiber is.

- Butter – Who doesn't care for their heated potato bested with a tablespoon of spread? I sure do!

- Parsley is for embellish

STEP BY STEP INSTRUCTIONS TO MAKE AIR FRYER BAKED POTATOES

1. Set your air fryer to 400 degrees.

2. Prick a few openings in the potatoes with a fork and shower the potato with cooking splash. Spot the potatoes in the air fryer bushel and close it.

3. Set the ideal opportunity for 30 minutes. After that, test the heated potato to check whether it was finished by checking how delicate the potato is. On the off chance that it isn't prepared at this point, place the potato back in for 10 minutes longer. Obviously, the time will differ contingent upon how huge your potatoes are. I utilized a medium measured reddish-brown potato for this.

4. Potatoes are prepared when their inside temperature arrives at 208 to 211° Fahrenheit. A fork effectively penetrates a bread cook when it's set. In the event that the potato is hard, heat somewhat more. Be that as it may, keep an eye out for over-preparing, or drying of the underskin will happen.

FIXINGS FOR AIR FRYER BAKED POTATOES

At the point when I worked at an office, Thursdays would consistently be considered treat day, and prepared potatoes were famous for bringing on the grounds that you can keep them warm in the simmering pot. The individual in control would consistently have various fixings to add to the highest point of the heated potato. Consistently it was somebody unique, so a similar individual didn't need to bring treats each day. We had a gathering of around 9 individuals doing this. I've made taco prepared potatoes that are likewise acceptable.

- Gorgonzola and wild ox sauce, acrid cream, green onions

- Sour cream, salsa, and chives

- Cottage cheddar, chives, and naturally ground pepper
- Leftover Instant Pot BBQ Chicken
- Leftover Zero Point Turkey Chili
- Leftover Taco fixings
- Broccoli and Nacho cheddar sauce, for example, Tostitos Medium Con Queso Sauce

THE CRISPY BREADED PORK AND CHOPS IN THE AIR FRYER

PREP TIME:10 mins

COOK TIME:12 mins

All out TIME:22 mins

YIELD:6

COURSE: Dinner

CUISINE: American

These Crispy Boneless Breaded Pork Chops turn out clammy within and crispy outwardly.

Fixings

- olive oil splash
- 6 3/4-inch thick focus cut boneless pork hacks, fat cut (5 oz each)
- kosher salt
- 1 huge egg, beaten
- 1/2 cup panko pieces, check names for GF
- 1/3 cup squashed cornflakes pieces
- 2 tbsp ground parmesan cheddar, exclude for dairy-free
- 1 1/4 tsp sweet paprika

- 1/2 tsp garlic powder
- 1/2 tsp onion powder
- 1/4 tsp stew powder
- 1/8 tsp dark pepper

Directions

1. Pre-heat the air fryer to 400F for 12 min. and delicately splash the container with oil.
2. Season pork hacks on the two sides with 1/2 tsp legitimate salt.
3. Combine panko, cornflake morsels, parmesan cheddar, 3/4 tsp genuine salt, paprika, garlic powder, onion powder, bean stew powder, and dark pepper in a huge shallow bowl.
4. Place the beaten egg in another. Plunge the pork into the egg, at that point scrap blend.
5. When the air fryer is prepared, place 3 of the slashes into the readied bin and spritz the top with oil.
6. Cook 12 minutes are turning midway, spritzing the two sides with oil. Put in a safe spot and rehash with the remaining.

Serving: 1pork slash, Calories: 378kcal, Carbohydrates: 8g, Protein: 33g, Fat: 13g, Cholesterol: 121mg, Sodium: 373mg, Sugar: 1g

Blue Smart Points:7

Green Smart Points:7

Purple Smart Points:7

Focuses +:7

AIR FRYER GRILLED CHEESE

Fixings

2 cuts of bread, for example, Village Hearth Light Italian

1 cut of Velveeta Original flavor cheddar item cuts

Cooking Spray or I Can't Believe It's Not Butter Spray.

Guidelines

Spot cheddar between two cuts of bread and spot the sandwich in your air fryer container. You can decide to splash each side of the bread before you put it in the crate. However, I like to shower the bread in the air fryer bin and afterward flip it to the opposite side and splash it once more.

Set your air fryer to 350 degrees and close the container. Set the clock to 5 minutes. Flip and afterward cook the opposite side for 3 minutes.

AIR FRYER STEAK

Air Fryer Steak – These steaks are also keto, low carb, and Weight Watcher well disposed. Serve them with some squashed cauliflower and green beans as an afterthought. I even have a convenient guide for making sense of temperatures and times for different cuts of steak below.

Directions

1. If your air-fryer requires preheating, preheat your air fryer.

2. Set the temperature to 400 degrees Fahrenheit.

3. Add Season to your steak with salt and pepper on each side.

4. Place the steak in your air fryer crate. Try not to cover the steaks. Set the opportunity to 12 minutes and flip the steak at 6. Present with vegetables or crushed cauliflower. This will give you a medium uncommon steak.

NOTES

Steak time can be very contingent upon what size it is.

- Category: Dinner
- Method: Air Fryer
- Cuisine: American

NUTRITION

- Serving Size: 4oz
- Calories: 250

- Sodium: 60
- Fat: 17
- Saturated Fat: 7
- Carbohydrates: 0
- Fiber: 0
- Protein: 23

AIR FRYER CHOCOLATE CAKE

Fixings

- 1 Perfect Size Duncan Hines Chocolate Lover's Cake

Guidelines

1. Preheat your air fryer 250 degrees. Follow the bundle headings for the cake blend and empty the hitter into the cake dish that accompanies the bundle. Addition the cake skillet into the air fryer container and set the clock to 20 minutes. Test the cake to check whether it is finished with a toothpick and in the event that it isn't cooked the cake for somewhat more.

THIN AIR FRYER BUFFALO CHICKEN WINGS

Fixings

- 1 pound of the cooked chicken wing(s) with skin and bone
- 1/2 cup of wild ox wing sauce
- 1/2 parcel shrouded valley farm flavoring

Directions

1. Putt the chicken wings in the air fryer bushel and set the temp to 400 degrees F and set the clock to 20 minutes

2. After the 20 minutes are done, take the chicken wings out and place them in a medium bowl. Add the farm flavoring blend to the chicken and hurl the wings to cover with the farm flavoring. Include the bison sauce and keep on hurling the chicken wings in the bowl until everything is very much covered.

NOTES

6 keen focuses for 1 wing.

NUTRITION

- Calories: 105
- Sugar: 0
- Sodium: 503mg
- Fat: 7
- Saturated Fat: 1
- Carbohydrates: 0
- Fiber: 0
- Protein: 10

AIR FRYER CHIMICHANGAS

Fixings

For the Chicken:

- 4 cups of store style cooked destroyed rotisserie chicken or destroyed chicken bosom
- 1 enormous onion, finely slashed
- 1 4oz. can slash green chilies
- 4 tbsp universally handy flour

- ¼ tsp garlic powder
- 1 tsp ground cumin

8 (6 in) flour tortillas

Garnishes for Chimichangas (discretionary)

- Reduced-Fat Cheddar Cheese
- Plain Greek Yogurt
- Cilantro or Scallions

Guidelines

1. Preheat air fryer to 400°F. Coat an enormous skillet with a cooking shower.

2. Add onions and green chilies to skillet and saute for 2 minutes. At the point when the onions are delicate, include flour, salt, cumin, garlic powder, enchilada sauce, and keep blending. At the point when the sauce has thickened, include precooked destroyed chicken. In the event that the sauce looks too thick, include some chicken stock to thin it out. (2 tablespoons to begin)

3. Take off heat and start setting up the chimichangas for cooking them in the air fryer.

4. Assemble chimichangas by spooning around 1/2 cup of the chicken blend onto every tortilla; overlap insides and move up.

5. Shower the outside of each filled tortilla with a cooking sprinkle; place 4 in the canister of air fryer, creaseside down. Cook 2 to 3 minutes or until delicately sautéed and warmed through. Repeat with remaining 4 filled tortillas.

- Category: Dinner
- Method: Air Fry
- Cuisine: Mexican

NUTRITION

- Serving Size: 1 chimichanga
- Calories: 311
- Sugar: 3
- Sodium: 374
- Fat: 7
- Saturated Fat: 1
- Carbohydrates: 20

- Fiber: 2
- Protein: 43

AIR FRYER HARD BOILED EGGS

Portrayal

Air Fryer Hard Boiled Eggs – are so natural you'll never make them on your stovetop again.

Fixings

- 6 enormous eggs (cold)

Guidelines

1. Set your wire rack that accompanied your air fryer inside the bin and spots the eggs over the wire rack. In the event that your air fryer didn't accompany a wire rack, at that point, simply place them in the base of the air fryer bin. I've done it with and without that, and the two methods work. I simply find that the wire rack is simpler to lift them the full scale of the crate without a moment's delay.

2. Set the temp to 250 and the clock to 16 minutes. After the eggs are done in the air fryer takes them out and puts them in an ice-water shower to stop the cooking. Strip the eggs

NOTES

- Blue Points: 0
- Green Points: 2
- Purple Points: 0
- Category: Appetizer
- Method: Air Fry
- Cuisine: American

NUTRITION

- Serving Size: 1 enormous egg
- Calories: 77

- Sugar: 0g
- Sodium: 62mg
- Fat: 5g
- Saturated Fat: 1.6g
- Carbohydrates: .6g
- Fiber: 0g
- Protein: 6.3g

Whiskey Bacon Burger

- PREP TIME: 10 m
- COOK TIME: 25 m
- TOTAL TIME: 35 m
- SERVINGS: 2

Fixings

- 1 TABLESPOON whiskey
- 2 TABLESPOONS dark colored sugar
- 3 strips maple bacon cut down the middle
- ¾ POUND ground hamburger 80% lean
- 1 TABLESPOON minced onion
- 2 TABLESPOONS BBQ sauce
- ½ TEASPOON salt
- freshly ground dark pepper
- 2 SLICES Colby Jack cheddar or Monterey Jack
- 2 Kaiser rolls

- lettuce and tomato for serving
- Zesty Burger Sauce:
- 2 TABLESPOONS BBQ sauce
- 2 TABLESPOONS mayonnaise
- ¼ TEASPOON ground paprika
- freshly ground dark pepper

Guidelines

1. Preheat the air fryer to 390ºF and empty a little water into the base of the air fryer cabinet. (This will help forestall the oil that dribbles into the base cabinet from consuming and smoking.)

2. Combine the whiskey and darker sugar in a little bowl. Spot the bacon strips in the air fryer crate and brush with the dark-colored sugar blend. Air-fry at 390ºF for 4 minutes. Flip the bacon over, brush with progressively darker sugar, and air-fry at 390ºF for an extra 4 minutes until crispy.

3. While the bacon is cooking, consolidate the ground hamburger, onion, BBQ sauce, salt, and pepper in a huge bowl. Combine all together with your hands and shape the meat into 2 patties.

4. Transfer the burger to the air fryer crate and air-fry the burgers at 370ºF for 15 to 20 minutes, contingent upon how you like your burger cooked (15 minutes for uncommon to medium-uncommon; 20 minutes for well-done). Flip the burgers over part of the way through the cooking procedure.

5. While the burgers are air-singing, make the burger sauce by consolidating the BBQ sauce, mayonnaise, paprika, and crisply ground dark pepper to taste in a bowl.

6. When the burgers are cooked exactly as you would prefer, top every patty with a cut of Colby Jack cheddar and air-fry for an extra moment, just to soften the cheddar. (You should stick the cheddar cut to the burger with a toothpick to keep it from blowing off in your air fryer.) Spread the sauce within the Kaiser moves, place the burgers on the moves, top with the whiskey bacon, lettuce, and tomato and appreciate!

Best Ever Air Fryer Hot Dog

You can make tasty franks in your air fryer. They taste simply like they were cooked on the flame broil.

Catchphrase: Air fryer Hot Dog, Air Fryer Recipes, How to Cook a Hot Dog in an Air Fryer

Planning Time: 3 minutes

Cook Time: 7 minutes

Absolute Time: 10 minutes

Servings: 2

Calories: 289kcal

Fixings

- 2 wieners
- 2 wiener buns
- 2 tablespoons ground cheddar whenever wanted

Directions

- Pre-heat the air fryer to 390 deg. for around 4 minutes. Spot two wieners into the air fryer, cook for around 5 minutes. Expel the sausage from the air fryer. Spot the wiener on a bun, include cheddar whenever wanted. Spot dressed wiener into the air fryer, and cook for an extra 2 minutes.

NUTRITION

Calories: 289kcal | Carbohydrates: 29g | Protein: 12g | Fat: 13g | Saturated Fat: 5g | Cholesterol: 36mg | Sodium: 613mg | Potassium: 119mg | Fiber: 0g | Sugar: 2g | Vitamin A: 150IU | Vitamin C: 0.6mg | Calcium: 193mg | Iron: 2.6mg

Cinnamon Rolls

- PREP TIME: 20 m
- COOK TIME: 9 m
- TOTAL TIME: 29 m
- SERVINGS:

-

Fixings

- 1 POUND solidified bread batter, defrosted
- ¼ CUP spread, liquefied and cooled
- ¾ CUP dark colored sugar
- 1½ TABLESPOONS ground cinnamon,

CREAM CHEESE GLAZE

- 4 OUNCES cream cheddar, mollified
- 2 TABLESPOONS spread, mellowed
- 1¼ CUPS powdered sugar
- ½ TEASPOON vanilla

Directions

1. Let the bread batter come to room temperature on the counter. On a gently floured surface, fold the batter into a 13-inch by 11-inch square shape. Position the square shape, so the 13-inch side is confronting you. Brush the softened spread everywhere throughout the batter, leaving a 1-inch outskirt revealed along the edge most remote away from you.

2. Combine the dark-colored sugar and cinnamon in a little bowl. Sprinkle the blend equitably over the buttered batter, keeping the 1-inch fringe revealed. Fold the batter into a log beginning with the edge nearest to you. Roll the mixture firmly, making a point to move equally and push out any air pockets. At the point when you find a workable pace edge of the mixture, press the batter onto the move to seal it together.

3. Cut the sign into 8 pieces, cutting slowly with a sawing movement, so you don't smooth the mixture. Turn the cuts on their sides and spread with a perfect kitchen towel. Let the moves sit in the hottest piece of your kitchen for 1½ to 2 hours to rise.

4. To make the coating, place the cream cheddar and spread in a microwave-safe bowl. Relax the blend in the microwave for 30 seconds one after another until it is anything but difficult to mix. Progressively include the powdered sugar and mix to join. Include the vanilla concentrate and speed until smooth. Put in a safe spot.

5. When the rolls have risen, pre-heat the air fryer to 350°F.

6. Transfer 4 of the moves to the air fryer bushel. Air-fry for 5 minutes. Turn the turns over and air-fry for an additional 4 minutes. Rehash with the staying 4 rolls.

7. Let the moves cool for two or three minutes before coating. Spread enormous dabs of cream cheddar coat over the warm cinnamon rolls, allowing a portion of the coating to trickle down the side of the rolls. Serve warm.

Air Fryer Jalapeno Poppers - A delectable sans gluten nibble

These Air Fryer Jalapeno Poppers are truly stunning. They are a zesty, mouth-watering, normally sans gluten nibble! We likewise offer up conventional oven directions as well!

Prep Time10 mins

Cook Time8 mins

Complete Time18 mins

Course: Appetizer

Cooking: American

Catchphrase: air fryer jalapeno poppers, jalapeno poppers

Servings: 4 individuals

Calories: 951kcal

Creator: Cindy Gordon (Vegetarian Mamma)

Fixings

- 10 jalapeno peppers split and deseeded
- 8 oz of cream cheddar I utilized a without dairy cream cheddar
- 1/4 c new parsley
- 3/4 c without gluten tortilla or bread pieces

Directions

1. Mix together 1/2 of pieces and cream cheddar. When consolidated, include the parsley.

2. Stuff each pepper with this blend.

3. Gently press the highest points of the peppers into the staying 1/4 c of pieces to make the top covering.

4. Cook in an air-fryer at 370 deg. F for 6-8 minutes.

Notes

- Remove every one of the seeds and white layer (except if you like things hot!)
- Wear gloves or be cautious in the wake of cutting.

Air Fryer Hot Dogs

Air Fryer Hot Dogs will be your preferred method to get ready wieners this late spring! Franks in the air fryer is tasty and simple to get ready.

Cook Time4 mins

All out Time4 mins

Course: Main Course

Food: American

Watchword: Air Fryer Hot Dogs

Servings: 4 individuals

Calories: 50kcal

Creator: Cindy Gordon

Gear

- Air Fryer

Fixings

- 4 Hot Dogs I utilized Veggie Dogs

Directions

1. Place franks into the air fryer bushel.

2. Cook franks in the air fryer at 390 degrees F for 4-5 minutes.

3. Put frank into a bun, top with your preferred sauces, and appreciate!

Notes

Air Fryer Hot Dog Tips:

- Depending on the "hound" you are utilizing to make this air fryer sausage formula, the canine may be somewhat oily. On the off chance that it is, that may cause some additional smoke with your air fryer.

- You can utilize this air fryer sausage system with a veggie-lover, vegan, or meat franks.

- You can cut exceptionally little cuts in the pooch of your canine to assist it with cooking all the more equitably and not extend or blow up during cooking. This is particularly useful with veggie hounds.

- You have the choice of additionally tossing in the buns while cooking your air fryer sausages. This assists with mellowing and warm the buns. I normally put mine in during the last 1-2 minutes.

Nutrition

Calories: 50kcal | Carbohydrates: 4g | Protein: 7g | Fat: 1g | Sodium: 430mg | Fiber: 1g | Sugar: 2g | Iron: 2mg

Air Fryer Meatloaf

Air Fryer Meatloaf is a distinct advantage. You can make the meatloaf in the air fryer a lot speedier than a conventional oven. You are going to adore this air fryer meatloaf formula.

Prep Time15 mins

Cook Time35 mins

Resting Time10 mins

Absolute Time1 hr

Course: Main Course

Cooking: American

Servings: 6 individuals

Calories: 317kcal

Creator: Cindy Gordon | Vegetarian Mamma

Gear

- Air Fryer

Fixings

- 1 lb Protein I utilized Beyond Meat, you can utilize hamburger, turkey, pork, and so on
- 2 T ketchup
- 1/2 cup onion diced
- 1 egg whisked
- 1 T mustard
- 1 T fluid smoke
- 1 t garlic powder
- 1/2 t salt
- 1/2 t smoked paprika
- 1/2 t oregano

Coating

- 1/4 c ketchup
- 1/4 c darker sugar
- 2 t Dijon mustard

Guidelines

1. The procedure is fundamentally a dump and mix. The things can be included in any request.

2. Add the breadcrumbs. Overlap in the onions. Include the flavors.

3. Pour in the crisp diced parsley. Include the fried egg. Pour in the ketchup, mustard, and fluid smoke. Mix well to consolidate.

4. Shape blend into a portionshape.

5. Air-Fry for 20 minutes at 370 deg. F.

6. Remove the air fryer crate from the unit. Combine the coating fixings. Spread the coating over the air fryer meatloaf.

7. keep cooking at a similar temperature for 10-15 minutes. (I you are utilizing meat, it needs to arrive at 165 degrees F least, utilize your meat thermometer).

8. Let air fryer meatloaf stop for 10 minutes. This will assist the fixings with unifying, and it will help when you go to cut it.

Air Fryer Meatloaf Tips:

- You can add vegetables to this formula. Decent augmentations are a ½ of diced carrots or ¾ c of diced chime pepper. On the off chance that you appreciate mushrooms, you can likewise add those to your air fryer meatloaf. Simply be certain that you diced them exceptionally little, so they cook through.

- If you need to make Paleo Meatloaf, you can sub out the breadcrumbs and sub in cassava flour or almond flour.

- Do not SKIP the "resting" some portion of this air fryer meatloaf formula. You have to allow the meatloaf to sit and rest to chill off. This will assist you with cutting into the air fryer meatloaf.

- Use a serrated blade to cut your air fryer meatloaf into cuts. This kind of blade will push the meatloaf .to not break separated when cutting.

- You need to beware of your air fryer meatloaf now and then. You have to check to ensure it isn't crisping excessively quick or consuming. If you feel that the highest point of your air fryer meatloaf is beginning to consume, you can put foil over the meatloaf to help with that. Be cautious that you secure the foil, so it doesn't fly out of sight fryer's heating zone.

- Don't attempt to surge this air fryer meatloaf formula by expanding the temperature. Cooking at a lower temperature assists with keeping the meatloaf soggy.

- Cooking times may shift a bit of relying upon how you shape your portion.

Nutrition

Calories: 317kcal | Carbohydrates: 15g | Protein: 64g | Fat: 4g | Saturated Fat: 1g | Cholesterol: 27mg | Sodium: 1110mg | Potassium: 130mg | Fiber: 5g | Sugar: 2g | Vitamin A: 147IU | Vitamin C: 1mg | Calcium: 161mg | Iron: 12mg

Air Fryer Fried Rice

Air Fryer Fried Rice is a speedy and simple air fryer formula. No compelling reason to arrange take out. This air fryer fried rice will satisfy your belly without the problem of additional oil and salt!

Prep Time5 mins

Cook Time15 mins

All out Time20 mins

Course: Side Dish

Food: Asian

Watchword: air fryer fried rice, fried rice

Servings: 4 individuals

Calories: 618kcal

- Air Fryer

Fixings

- 3 c rice cooked and cold
- 1 c solidified vegetables I utilized carrot, corn, broccoli, and edamame
- 1/3 c coconut aminos
- 1 T oil
- 2 eggs mixed (discretionary)

Guidelines

1. To make your air fryer fried rice, put your virus rice into an enormous bowl.

2. Then add your solidified vegetables to the rice bowl.

3. If you are utilizing egg or another protein, add it to the rice bowl now.

4. Next up, you are going to include the coconut aminos and oil to your bowl.

5. Mix, blend, blend until very much joined. At that point, move to the rice blend to an oven-safe holder.

6. Place that holder into your air fryer. Cook the air fryer fried rice at 360 degrees F for 15 minutes. I would propose blending multiple times through the 15 minutes.

7. Enjoy!

Notes

Tips for Air Fryer Fried Rice:

- Add in whatever protein you like: eggs, tofu, chicken, turkey

- Be sure to mix the air fryer fried rice a few times inside the brief cooking time frame. This encourages it to cook equitably.

- If you are without gluten, make certain to check the soy sauce on the off chance that you are utilizing that. Coconut Aminos is my without gluten go to with regards to a soy sauce season.

- Use any mixes of solidified veggies that you like.

What to present with Air Fryer Fried Rice:

- Crispy Tofu

- Sheet Pan Lemon Tofu

- Sweet Thai Chili Tofu

Nutrition

Calories: 618kcal | Carbohydrates: 121g | Protein: 14g | Fat: 7g | Saturated Fat: 1g | Cholesterol: 82mg | Sodium: 512mg | Potassium: 286mg | Fiber: 4g | Sugar: 1g | Vitamin A: 2429IU | Vitamin C: 5mg | Calcium: 63mg | Iron: 2mg

Air Fryer Broccoli

Air Fryer Broccoli is a heavenly and simple to make air fryer formula. You will begin to look all starry eyed at all over again with this air fried broccoli!

Prep Time2 mins

Cook Time10 mins

Complete Time12 mins

Course: Side Dish

Cooking: American

Catchphrase: air fryer broccoli

Servings: 2 individuals

Calories: 25kcal

Creator: Cindy Gordon

Fixings

- 3 c broccoli florets
- 1 t oil
- salt and pepper to taste

Directions

1. To make your air fryer broccoli, tenderly hurl the cut broccoli florets with the oil. Season with salt and pepper.

2. Place broccoli into air fryer bushel.

3. Turn on the air fryer to 300 degrees F for 10 minutes. Shake air fryer bushel following 5 minutes.

4. ENJOY your air fryer broccoli!

Notes

In the event that you like to a greater degree a roasted sort of broccoli, you can cook for 1-2 minutes longer.

If you lean toward progressively delicate broccoli, you can cook for 1-2 minutes less.

Nutrition

Calories: 25kcal | Carbohydrates: 1g | Fat: 2g | Sodium: 5mg | Potassium: 52mg | Vitamin A: 105IU | Vitamin C: 14.7mg | Calcium: 8mg | Iron: 0.1mg

Air Fryer Potato Pancakes

The Air Fryer Potato Pancakes are crispy, yet delicate and will fulfill everybody's tastebuds. This potato flapjacks formula can be filled in as a primary side or side dish.

Prep Time10 mins

Cook Time10 mins

Absolute Time20 mins

Course: Appetizer, Side Dish

Cooking: American

Catchphrase: remaining crushed potato hotcakes, potato flapjacks

Servings: 6 individuals

Calories: 12kcal

Creator: Cindy Gordon | Vegetarian Mamma

Gear

- Air Fryer

Fixings

- 2 1/3 c remaining pureed potatoes cold
- 3 green onions diced (whites and greens)
- 1 t oregano
- 1 t smoked paprika
- 2 T All-reason without gluten flour OR AP Flour

Directions

1. To make potato flapjacks, scoop the extra pureed potatoes into a bowl.

2. Then include the diced green onions (scallions) to your crushed potato bowl.

3. Pour the flour and flavors into the bowl.

4. Scramble one egg in a little bowl at that point add it to the potato bowl blend.

5. Mix all fixings well. Form into patties. Put the potato flapjacks into the air fryer bushel.
6. Plate your potato hotcakes and present with a side of acrid cream (discretionary).

Notes

Tips for Leftover pounded potato flapjacks:

- You can utilize pureed potatoes, ground potatoes, or hashbrowns favor pureed potatoes. Master Tip: on the off chance that you utilized ground potatoes, you should press the water from them. IOn the off chance that they are too watery, this will influence the potato hotcakes formula.

- If you need your potato hotcakes crispy, make them more slender.

- If the surface is an issue, you can mix all fixings in a food processor to get a smooth surface for your potato flapjacks.

- Be cautious flipping over the potato flapjacks in the air fryer bushel, and they will be fragile.

- Be cautious when plating, if the potato hotcakes are dropped, they will break separated.

- ProTip: If you need your remaining squashed potato hotcakes to be brilliant darker, you can spritz some oil on them.

Cinnamon Rolls with Cream Cheese Glaze

- PREP TIME: 25 m

- COOK TIME: 30 m

- TOTAL TIME: 55 m

- SERVINGS:

+

-

Fixings

- 1 POUND solidified bread batter, defrosted Cinnamon Roll Dough formula, see here,
- ¼ CUP spread dissolved and cooled
- ¾ CUP dark colored sugar
- 1½ TABLESPOONS ground cinnamon

CREAM CHEESE GLAZE

- 4 OUNCES cream cheddar mellowed
- 2 TABLESPOONS spread mollified
- 1¼ CUPS powdered sugar
- ½ TEASPOON vanilla

Directions

1. Let the batter come to room temperature on the counter. On a softly floured surface, fold the mixture into a 16-inch by 13-inch square shape. Position the square shape, so the shorter 13-inch side is confronting you. Brush the softened margarine over the batter, leaving a 1-inch outskirt revealed along the edge most remote away from you.

2. Combine the dark-colored sugar and cinnamon in a little bowl. Sprinkle the blend equitably over the buttered mixture, keeping the 1-inch fringe revealed. Fold the batter into a log beginning with the edge nearest to you. Roll the batter firmly, making a point to move equally and push out any air pockets. At the point when you find a good pace edge of the batter, press the mixture onto the move to seal it together.

3. Cut the log of batter into 12 pieces, cutting slowly with a sawing movement, so you don't smooth the mixture. Turn the cuts on their sides on a lubed and lined (with silicone or material) 9" x 13" sheet container and spread with a spotless kitchen towel. Let the moves sit in the hottest piece of your kitchen for an hour to rise.

4. To make the coating, place the cream cheddar and margarine in a microwave-safe bowl. Relax the blend in the microwave for 30 seconds one after another until it is anything but

difficult to mix. Bit by bit includes the powdered sugar and mix to join. Include the vanilla concentrate and rush until smooth. Put in a safe spot.

5. Air-Fryer Directions: When the rolls have risen, pre-heat the air fryer to 350°F. Move 6 of the moves to the air fryer bin. Air-fry for 5 minutes. Turn the turns over and air-fry for an additional 4 minutes. Rehash with the rest of the rolls.

6. Oven Baking Directions: Pre-heat the oven to 375°F. Move the sheet container to the oven and heat the moves for 25 – 30 minutes, or until daintily cooked. Spread with foil if the moves begin to get excessively darker.

7. Let the moves cool for a few minutes before coating. Spread huge dabs of cream cheddar coat over the warm cinnamon rolls, allowing a portion of the coating to dribble down the side of the rolls. Serve warm and appreciate it!

Sweet Chocolate Berry Sandwich

- PREP TIME: 5 m
- COOK TIME: 6 m
- TOTAL TIME: 11 m
- SERVINGS: 4

Fixings

- 8 SLICES cinnamon raisin bread
- ½ CUP chocolate hazelnut spread
- ½ CUP raspberry jam
- 24 raspberries
- 1 TABLESPOON Butter mollified

Directions

1. Spread the spread on one side of each of the 8 cuts of bread. Amass the sandwiches by putting the bread cuts margarine side down on a work surface. Separation and spread the chocolate hazelnut spread on four of the cuts of bread. Gap and spread the raspberry jam on the other four cuts of bread. Press the raspberries into the four cuts of chocolate secured bread, and top with the jam secured cuts.

2. FPre-heat a skillet or frying pan (in a perfect world square fit as a fiddle) over medium heat. Include the amassed sandwiches and fry on the two sides until pleasantly seared – around 3 to 4 minutes. Appreciate with a tall glass of milk!

Monte Cristo Bread Pudding

- PREP TIME: 15 m
- COOK TIME: 35 m
- RESTING TIME: 20 m
- TOTAL TIME: 1 h 10 m
- SERVINGS: 8

Fixings

- 12 OUNCES craftsman sourdough bread cut into 3D shapes (around 6 cups)
- 6 eggs
- 2 CUPS cream
- 2 TEASPOONS vanilla concentrate
- 1 TABLESPOON Dijon mustard
- ½ TEASPOON salt
- 1 CUP diced ham
- 1½ CUPS cooked diced turkey
- 8 OUNCES Swiss cheddar ground
- powdered sugar
- raspberry jam for serving

Directions

1. Pre-heat the oven to 350°F. Oil 8 individual 1 cup ramekins with spread and spot them on a heating sheet.

2. Cut the portion of bread into enormous 3D shapes and spot the solid shapes in a huge bowl.

3. Include the vanilla concentrate, Dijon mustard and salt.

4. Add the ham, turkey and Swiss cheddar to the bowl with the bread 3D shapes and hurl to join everything. Pour the egg custard over top and delicately hurl to cover all the bread solid shapes. Let the blend lay on the counter for 20 minutes.

5. Stir the blend again and spoon it uniformly into the readied ramekins.

6. Transfer the heating sheet with filled ramekins to the oven.

7. Dust with some powdered sugar and serve quickly with some raspberry jam dolloped on top.

Zesty Black Bean Turkey Burgers with Cumin-Avocado Spread

- PREP TIME: 10 m
- COOK TIME: 20 m
- TOTAL TIME: 30 m
- SERVINGS: 2

Fixings

- 1 CUP canned dark beans depleted and flushed
- ¾ POUND ground turkey
- 2 TABLESPOONS minced red onion
- 1 Jalapeño pepper seeded and minced
- 2 TABLESPOONS plain breadcrumbs
- ½ TEASPOON salt
- ½ TEASPOON bean stew powder
- ¼ TEASPOON cayenne pepper
- olive or vegetable oil

- 2 SLICES pepper Jack cheddar
- toasted burger rolls cut tomatoes, lettuce leaves
- Cumin-Avocado Spread:
- 1 ready avocado
- juice of 1 lime
- 1 TEASPOON ground cumin
- ½ TEASPOON salt
- 1 TABLESPOON hacked new cilantro
- freshly ground dark pepper

Directions

1. Place the dark beans in a huge bowl and crush them somewhat with the rear of a fork. Include the ground turkey, red onion, Jalapeño pepper, breadcrumbs, salt, stew powder and cayenne pepper. Blend in with your hands to consolidate every one of the fixings and afterward shape them into 2 patties. Brush the two sides of the burger patties with a little olive or vegetable oil.

2. Pre-heat the air fryer to 380ºF.

3. Transfer the burgers to the air fryer bin and air-fry for 20 minutes, flipping them over part of the way through the cooking procedure. Top the burgers with the pepper Jack cheddar (protecting the cuts to the burgers with a toothpick) throughout the previous 2 minutes of the cooking procedure.

4. While the burgers are cooking, make the cumin avocado spread. Spot the avocado, lime juice, cumin and salt in food processor and procedure until smooth. (For a chunkier spread, you can pound this by turn in a bowl.) Stir in the cilantro and season with crisply ground dark pepper. Chill the spread until you are prepared to serve.

5. When the burgers have got done with cooking, expel them from the air fryer and let them lay on a plate, secured tenderly with aluminum foil. Brush a little olive oil on the internal parts of the burger rolls. Spot the moves, cut side up, into the air fryer bushel and air-fry at 400°F for 1 moment to toast and warm them.

6. Spread the cumin-avocado spread on the rolls and fabricate your burgers with lettuce and cut tomatoes and some other fixing you like. Serve warm with a side of sweet potato fries.

Air-Fried Pizza Burgers

- PREP TIME: 10 m
- COOK TIME: 15 m
- TOTAL TIME: 25 m
- SERVINGS: 4

Fixings

- 1 POUND meatloaf blend ground hamburger, veal and pork
- 1 TABLESPOON minced onion
- ⅓ CUP hacked pepperoni or scaled down pepperoni cuts
- 1 TABLESPOON tomato glue
- 1 TEASPOON Italian flavoring
- ½ TEASPOON salt
- freshly ground dark pepper
- 1 CUP pizza sauce
- 6 OUNCES cut mozzarella cheddar
- 4 dried up round moves crusty bread rolls or focaccia bread

Directions

1. Place the meatloaf blend, minced onion, pepperoni, tomato glue, Italian flavoring salt and pepper in a huge bowl. Blend altogether until all around joined. Separation the meat into 4 equivalent parts and afterward structure the cheeseburgers, being mindful so as not to over-handle the meat. One great approach to do this is to toss the meat to and fro between your hands like a baseball, pressing the meat each time you get it. Level the balls into patties, making a space or divot in the focal point of every party. This will help keep the burger level as it cooks.

2. Split the moves into equal parts and brush the cut side with a little olive oil.

3. Pre-heat the air fryer to 370°F.

4. Air-fry the burger for 15 minutes, flipping them over partially through the cooking time. Spoon a little pizza sauce on every burger and top with the cut mozzarella cheddar. Air-fry at 370°F for 3 additional minutes until the cheddar has softened.

6. Transfer the refreshed burgers to the toasted moves, sprinkle somewhat more Italian flavoring on top, and serve right away.

Skillet Pizza Dip

- PREP TIME: 20 m
- COOK TIME: 30 m
- TOTAL TIME: 50 m
- SERVINGS: 8

Fixings

- 8 OUNCES cream cheddar relaxed
- 1½ CUPS ground mozzarella cheddar isolated
- 1 TEASPOON Italian flavoring
- ½ TEASPOON garlic powder
- 1 POUND pizza mixture
- ½ CUP pizza sauce
- 1 TABLESPOON ground Parmesan cheddar
- 2 TABLESPOONS diced red and green ringer peppers
- 2 TABLESPOONS cut olives
- 2 TABLESPOONS diced or smaller than expected pepperoni
- ½ TEASPOON dried oregano
- olive oil

Guidelines

1. Pre-heat the oven to 375°F.

2. Combine the relaxed cream cheddar and one cup of the mozzarella cheddar in a little bowl. Include the Italian flavoring and garlic powder and blend well.

3. Cut the pizza mixture into 16 pieces. Fold each piece into a ball and spot the balls around the outside edge of an 11-inch non-stick sauté dish, leaving the focal point of the container unfilled.

4. Spread the cream cheddar blend into the focal point of the skillet. Spread the pizza sauce over the cheddar blend. Top with the remaining ½ cup of mozzarella cheddar and ground Parmesan cheddar. Disperse the diced peppers, olives, and pepperoni on top and sprinkle with the dried oregano.

5. Brush the batter balls with a little olive oil and prepare at 375°F for 30 minutes.

6. Transfer to an enormous plate and serve quickly, or wrap the handle with a kitchen towel and serve directly from the hot skillet.

Air Fryer Corn on the Cob

Air fryer old fashioned corn is the snappiest and most heavenly air fryer recipes to date. The air fryer rapidly roasts the sweet corn, new or solidified, into a powerful side dish! You are going to cherish this air fried fresh corn!

Prep Time2 mins

Cook Time8 mins

Complete Time10 mins

Course: Side Dish

Servings: 2 individuals

Calories: 61kcal

Creator: Cindy Gordon

Fixings

- 2 ears of new sweet corn husk and silk expelled, split

- 1 T oil
- salt and pepper to taste

Directions

1. Cut corn down the middle, so you have four pieces.

2. Gently pour 1 T of oil over corn and focus on with your hands. Spot corn parts into the air fryer crate.

3. Turn the air-fryer on to 380 degrees F and cook for 8 minutes. At the brief imprint, evacuate crate, shake, and come back to cooking.

4. When air fryer stops, expel corn cautiously from the crate (it will be HOT!) Slather with increasingly salt and pepper and spread on the off chance that you wish!

Air Fryer Jalapeno Poppers - A delightful sans gluten nibble

These Air Fryer Jalapeno Poppers are truly astounding. They are a hot, mouth-watering, normally sans gluten nibble! We likewise offer up customary oven guidelines as well!

Prep Time10 mins

Cook Time8 mins

Complete Time18 mins

Course: Appetizer

Cooking: American

Catchphrase: air fryer jalapeno poppers, jalapeno poppers

Servings: 4 individuals

Calories: 951kcal

Creator: Cindy Gordon (Vegetarian Mamma)

Fixings

- 10 jalapeno peppers split and deseeded

- 8 oz of cream cheddar I utilized a without dairy cream cheddar
- 1/4 c new parsley
- 3/4 c without gluten tortilla or bread pieces

Directions

1. Mix together 1/2 of pieces and cream cheddar. When joined, including the parsley.
2. Stuff each pepper with this blend.
3. Gently press the highest points of the peppers into the staying 1/4 c of morsels to make the top covering.
4. PCook in an air fryer at 370 degrees F for 6-8 minutes OR in a regular roven at 375 degrees F for 20 minutes.
5. Let cool and ENJOY!

Notes

- Remove every one of the seeds and white film (except if you like things hot!)
- Wear gloves or be cautious subsequent to ecutting and deseeding these jalapenos.

pareNutrition

Calories: 951kcal | Carbohydrates: 83g | Protein: 23g | Fat: 69g | Saturated Fat: 22g | Sodium: 890mg | Potassium: 430mg | Fiber: 21g | Sugar: 14g | Vitamin A: 2773IU | Vitamin C: 186mg | Calcium: 184mg | Iron: 4mg

Air Fryer Risotto Balls (otherwise known as arancini balls)

Game-changing air fryer risotto balls to attempt at the present time! We love our simple to make air fryer recipes! Utilize your remaining risotto to make these flavorful arancini balls!

Prep Time20 mins

Cook Time10 mins

Complete Time30 mins

Course: Appetizer

Catchphrase: air fryer risotto balls

Servings: 8 individuals

Calories: 264kcal

Fixings

Risotto

- 1 T olive oil
- 1 cup onions diced exceptionally little
- 4 cups vegetable soup
- 1 cup arborio rice
- 1 cup parmesan cheddar

Breading

- 1.5 cups Bread Crumbs I utilized Ian's GF Italian Panko
- 2 eggs beaten

Directions

1. If utilizing remaining risotto, jump to stage 6.

2. Add olive oil to a profound and huge pot over medium heat. Heat the oil. Add the onions and saute until delicate.

3. Add dry rice and saute for 1 moment.

4. Next, include 2 cups of veggie stock. Let the soup cook down while you persistently mix to maintain a strategic distance from any consumption. When the fluid has been cooked down, include 2 additional cups. Proceed with this procedure until all your fluid is ingested, and your rice is delicate. This procedure should take around 20 minutes. Mix in parmesan.

5. Pour risotto into a goulash dish or sheet skillet. Cool for 1-2 hours in the ice chest. (This progression is significant. The risotto HAS to be cold to have the option to be folded into balls).

6. In a little bowl, place the bread scraps. In another bowl, place the beaten eggs.

7. Remove chilled risotto (rice blend) from the ice chest. Fold into 1-inch rice balls. Dunk into eggs then into bread pieces to cover the whole ball. Do this until you come up short on fixings.

8. Place folded and covered balls again into the cooler for 45 minutes.

9. Remove from ice chest and spot into Air Fryer in little clumps. The balls are really done around minute 6-7 however the searing doesn't occur until minute 8-10

Air Fryer Green Beans

Air Fryer Green Beans will be the ideal expansion to your develop assortment of tasty air fryer recipes! In the event that you love green beans, this is a brisk and delectable approach to make them!

Prep Time2 mins

Cook Time10 mins

Absolute Time12 mins

Course: Side Dish

Cooking: American

Catchphrase: air fryer green beans, air fryer recipes

Servings: 4 servings

Calories: 22kcal

Creator: Cindy Gordon

Fixings

- 2 c green beans
- 1/2 oil

Directions

1. Wash green beans and cut off finishes if vital. Hurl beans with oil.

2. Put beans into the air fryer. Cook It 390 deg. F for 10 minutes.

3. ENJOY.

Notes

I like my beans to have a tad of a crunch still, on the off chance that you might want your beans "progressively" all around done, cook 2-3 minutes longer.

Would i be able to utilize FROZEN green beans in my air fryer?

Indeed, you can! I know this on the grounds that the first occasion when I attempted it, my green beans were solidified yet in my refrigerator! Agh! The cooling cabinet broke down and got excessively cool!

Be that as it may, rather than quitting, I chose to attempt it. It worked. In the event that your beans are solidified and have some solidified dampness on them, they may feel somewhat more spongy when completely arranged. Be that as it may, they, despite everything, taste astonishing!

Gluten-Free Air Fryer Eggplant Parmesan

Gluten-Free Eggplant Parmesan is anything but difficult to make! This dish is prepared, not fried! We have included sans dairy and Vegan alternatives as well!

Prep Time35 mins

Cook Time10 mins

Absolute Time1 hr 5 mins

Course: Main Course

Food: Italian

Watchword: air fryer recipes, eggplant parmesan

Servings: 4 individuals

Calories: 449kcal

Creator: Cindy Gordon (Vegetarian Mamma)

Fixings

- 1 10 oz box spaghetti I utilized a gluten-free kind
- 2 cup of your preferred marinara sauce
- 1 medium eggplant
- 2 eggs
- 1.5 cups sans gluten panko pieces
- 1/3 c parmesan cheddar discretionary
- 1 T Italian Seasoning
- 1 cup mozzarella cheddar destroyed
- fresh basil and cilantro

Notes

Sans dairy choices are to preclude the parmesan, or you can utilize veggie-lover parmesan. For a vegetarian alternative, you can utilize maple syrup rather than eggs!

Contingent upon the size of your air fryer, you may need to set up this formula in clumps.

If your eggplant pieces are not getting brilliant darker, you can spritz them with shower oil to enable them to be fresh.

Air Fryer Brussel Sprouts

Air Fryer Brussel Sprouts is a straightforward and simple to make side dish. You will be astounded at the delightful air fryer vegetable recipes! If you are thinking about how to cook Brussel grows in the air fryer, we will educate you!

Prep Time5 mins

Cook Time10 mins

All out Time15 mins

Course: Side Dish

Food: American

Watchword: Air Fryer Brussel Sprouts

Servings: 4 individuals

Calories: 31kcal

Fixings

- 3 c divided Brussel grows
- 1 T olive oil
- 1/4 t salt
- 1/4 t pepper

Directions

1. Toss Brussel grows with olive and salt/pepper.
2. Place into an air fryer crate.
3. Set an air fryer for 400 degrees F and cook 8-12 minutes.

Notes

The most effective method to eat your Air Fryer Brussel Sprouts:

There are such a large number of ways that you can make the most of your air fryer Brussel grows. One of my new most loved ways is to hurl them with handcrafted prepared sauce. You can utilize the sauce formula here. (Snap here if on the web) You won't have to utilize all the sauce, simply spoon it on in limited quantities of a period until you arrive at your ideal level.

Who Would be able to use frozen Brussel sprouts

You can utilize solidified Brussels, and they will totally cook, anyway, you will lose a portion of the crunch factor! Have you attempted this? Drop me a note in the remarks!

Delicate OUTSIDE, BUT CHEWY INSIDE?

On the off chance that you like a milder Brussel all through, you can microwave the Brussels for a couple of moments before air fricasseeing. This will assist the general surface with being consistent. These Brussels turn out delicate outwardly and somewhat chewier within (as the formula is composed).

SPROUTS BURNING?

Be certain that you are cutting the sprouts in thirds or parts relying upon the size of the sprouts. The littler the pieces, the simpler they will consume. Anyway, the greater pieces won't cook the whole distance. It's a tad of a game. You can generally do a couple as a test cluster. Sprouts sizes can truly differ!

HOW DO I COOK WITHOUT AN AIR FRYER?

You can roast your Brussels at 425 degrees F for around 20 minutes! Mix once in the center of the time period!

Nutrition

Calories: 31kcal | Fat: 3g | Sodium: 145mg

Air Fryer Chickpeas

Air Fryer Chickpeas are a fast and flavorful air fryer nibble. You are going to cherish these irresistible air-fried garbanzo beans.

Prep Time2 mins

Cook Time15 mins

Complete Time17 mins

Course: Snack

Cooking: American

Catchphrase: air fryer chickpeas

Servings: 4 individuals

Calories: 205kcal

Fixings

- 15 oz Garbanzo Beans depleted and washed
- 1 T oil
- salt and pepper to taste

Directions

1. In a little bowl, blend the beans in with the oil.
2. Put beans into air fryer crate and cook at 390 degrees F for 15 minutes. Shake at the brief imprint. Shake again at the brief imprint and season with salt and pepper. Keep on cooking.
3. ENJOY!

Notes

If you incline toward a crispier chickpea, cook a touch longer. Have a go at cooking 1-2 minutes until you arrive at the fresh you need!

Nutrition

Calories: 205kcal | Carbohydrates: 29g | Protein: 9g | Fat: 6g | Sodium: 7mg | Potassium: 309mg | Fiber: 8g | Sugar: 5g | Vitamin A: 30IU | Vitamin C: 1.4mg | Calcium: 52mg | Iron: 3.1mg

Air Fryer Honey Sriracha Cauliflower

Air Fryer Honey Sriracha Cauliflower is a tasty hot air fryer formula finished off with a sweet and fiery Sriracha sauce. This veggie lover air fryer formula is a champ for game day!

Prep Time10 mins

Cook Time10 mins

Complete Time25 mins

Course: Main Course

Cooking: Thai

Catchphrase: air fryer, nectar sriracha cauliflower

Servings: 4 servings

Calories: 113kcal

Fixings

Sauce

- 1/3 c nectar
- 1/3 c Sriracha
- 1 T coconut aminos
- 1/4 t sesame seed oil
- 1 T rice vinegar

Vegetable

- 3-4 c cauliflower florets

Directions

1. In a bowl, combine the nectar, Sriracha, coconut aminos, sesame seed oil, and rice vinegar. Whisk together, put in a safe spot.

2. Dip every cauliflower piece into the sauce to cover the cauliflower with sauce.

3. Gently spot cauliflower in the air fryer at 370 degrees F for 10 minutes. Shake the bushel mid path through (about the brief imprint). 10 minutes will give you a delicate cauliflower. On the off chance that you lean toward crunchier cauliflower, decrease the time.

4. Top with extra sauce in the wake of plating.

Notes

- Serve with celery and farm or blue cheddar dressing as an afterthought for plunging.
- Save a couple of moments and purchase pre-washed, pre-sliced cauliflower for this formula to meet up considerably quicker!

Nutrition

Calories: 113kcal | Carbohydrates: 28g | Protein: 1g | Sodium: 637mg | Potassium: 267mg | Fiber: 1g | Sugar: 24g | Vitamin A: 30IU | Vitamin C: 51.2mg | Calcium: 16mg | Iron: 0.5mg

Air Fried Honey Mustard Pork Chops

- PREP TIME: 10 m
- COOK TIME: 15 m
- TOTAL TIME: 25 m
- SERVINGS: 2

Fixings

- 2 bone-in pork cleaves 1-inch thick
- ¼ CUP nectar
- 2 TABLESPOONS entire grain mustard
- 1 TEASPOON Worcestershire sauce
- 1 TABLESPOON new lemon juice
- ¼ TEASPOON smoked paprika
- olive oil
- 10 OUNCES Brussels grows split
- ¾ POUND smaller than usual gold potatoes divided
- salt and newly ground dark pepper

Directions

1. Combine the nectar, entire grain mustard, Worcestershire sauce, lemon squeeze, and smoked paprika in a medium-size meal dish. Include the pork slashes and penetrate openings in the hacks a few times and surrender the cleaves to cover with the marinade. On the off chance that conceivable, turn the pork slashes more than 1 or multiple times during the marinating time.

2. When prepared to air-fry, expel the pork slashes from the cooler and let them lay on the counter while you set up the vegetables.

3. Preheat the air fryer to 400°F.

4. Put the Brussels sprouts and potatoes in the air fryer bin. Shower with olive oil and season with salt and crisply ground dark pepper.

5. Move the vegetables to a bowl and spread with aluminum foil.

6. Place the pork cleaves in the air fryer crate and pour the marinade over the top. Air-fry for 10-12 minutes at 400ºF. The pork slashes should arrive at an interior temperature of 155°F with a moment read thermometer.

7. Transfer the slashes to a plate. Tent the slashes with aluminum foil to rest.

8. While the pork slashes are resting, return the Brussels sprouts and potatoes to the air fryer.

9. Plate the pork hacks and pour the sauce on the base of the air fryer crate over the pork cleaves. Present with vegetables as an afterthought.

Products of the soil Stuffed Pork Loin with Pineapple Glaze - Oven Method

- PREP TIME: 20 m
- COOK TIME: 1 h
- TOTAL TIME: 1 h 20 m
- SERVINGS: 4

Fixings

- 4 CUPS cubed Hawaiian sweet bread
- ⅓ CUP warm chicken stock
- ¼ CUP ground onion
- ½ CUP diced dried pineapple
- ½ CUP diced dried mango
- ½ TEASPOON dried sage
- 2 TABLESPOONS hacked crisp parsley
- 1 egg delicately beaten
- ⅓ CUP hacked blended nuts pistachios, cashews, walnuts, almonds, however no peanuts
- ½ TEASPOON salt

- freshly ground dark pepper
- 1 1/2 POUNDS pork midsection roast around 12 crawls long
- 8 OUNCES pineapple jam
- 1 TABLESPOON soy sauce
- 1 TABLESPOON dark colored sugar
- ½ head broccoli florets
- ½ head cauliflower florets
- olive oil

Directions

1. Preheat the oven to 425°F.

2. Make the stuffing by consolidating the bread 3D squares, warm chicken stock, and ground onion together in a bowl. Mix in the dried pineapple, mango, sage, parsley, egg, hacked nuts, salt, and naturally ground dark pepper. Join well.

3. Double butterfly the pork flank as follows. Spot the pork flank on a cutting board with one end pointing towards you. Utilizing a long cutting blade, make a cut into the pork flank corresponding to the cutting board and around 1/3 of the path from the top surface of the midsection. Stop before you cut totally through the midsection. Flip the pork midsection over with the goal that the remove side is from your blade and what was the base of the flank turns into the top. Make another entry point into the pork flank, corresponding to the cutting board and 1/3 of the path down from the top surface of the midsection. Stop before you cut totally through the flank. Open the folds of meat with the goal that the pork flank is presently a huge square shape multiple times its unique width.

4. Cover the pork with a bit of saran wrap and pound the meat gently with a meat hammer to an even thickness.

5. Season the pork with salt and naturally ground dark pepper. Spread the stuffing over the pork, leaving a 1-inch verge on one short end. Beginning from the opposite end, fold the pork into a log, jam move style. Tie the pork midsection with kitchen twine in 3 to 4 places down the roast to verify it, rub the outside of the roast with olive oil, and season it with salt and naturally ground dark pepper. Move the pork to an enormous roasting container.

6. P the dish to the oven and roast at 425°F for 20 minutes.

7. While the meat is cooking, make the coating by consolidating the pineapple jelly, dark colored sugar, and soy sauce in a bowl. Following 20 minutes of roasting, brush a portion of the coating over the pork flank. Include the broccoli and cauliflower florets around the roast, showering with olive oil and flavoring with salt and pepper. Roast for an extra 20 minutes, coating the pork two additional occasions during the cooking procedure. The pork should arrive at an interior temperature of 145°F to 155°F on a moment read thermometer embedded into the thickest piece of the flank.

8. Keep on roasting the vegetables for 5 additional minutes, until the vegetables are cooked exactly as you would prefer. Cut the pork into ½-inch cuts and present with the roasted vegetables.

Boursin Twice Baked Stuffed Potatoes

- PREP TIME: 15 m
- COOK TIME: 1 h 30 m
- TOTAL TIME: 1 h 45 m
- SERVINGS: 4

Fixings

- 5 huge reddish-brown potatoes
- olive oil
- 5.25 OUNCES Boursin® Garlic and Herb Cheese mellowed
- 4 TABLESPOONS unsalted spread
- 1 egg beaten
- ⅓ CUP cream
- 1 TEASPOON salt
- freshly ground dark pepper
- paprika
- fresh chives cleaved

Directions

1. Preheat the oven to 400°F.

2. Spot the potatoes on a heating sheet and prepare at 400°F for 60 minutes. Let the potatoes cool for at any rate 10 minutes.

3. Cut an oval into the highest point of four of the potatoes, leaving about ½-inch of the skin around the edge of every potato. Scoop out within the potato and spot it in a bowl. Add pieces to the bowl with the remainder of the potatoes. Pound the potatoes with a potato masher or utilize a potato ricer to squash the potatoes.

4. Add the Boursin® cheddar, margarine, egg, cream, and salt. Mix until very much consolidated and season with newly ground dark pepper.

5. Spoon the potato blend into the potato shells, heaping them high. Sprinkle the tops with a little paprika.

6. Bake at 375°F for 30 minutes. Topping with some cleaved crisp chives and serve right away.

Creamed Spinach Casserole

- PREP TIME: 15 m
- COOK TIME: 30 m
- TOTAL TIME: 45 m
- SERVINGS: 13

Fixings

- 20 OUNCES solidified cleaved spinach defrosted
- 16 OUNCES cream cheddar relaxed
- 1 CUP unsalted margarine mollified and isolated
- salt and naturally ground dark pepper
- 1½ CUPS breadcrumbs

Guidelines

1. Pre-heat the oven to 350°F and oil within a 3-quart goulash dish with the spread.

3. Whip the cream cheddar and ¾ cup of the margarine together in a bowl. Overlay in the spinach and season with salt and naturally ground dark pepper. Spread the blend into the readied goulash dish.

4. Melt the rest of the margarine and consolidate it with the breadcrumbs. Sprinkle the breadcrumbs over the spinach in the goulash dish and move the dish to the oven.

5. Bakefor 25 to 30 minutes until the blend is bubbly and the breadcrumbs are delicately sautéed. Let the meal rest for in any event 10 minutes before serving.

Brined Roast Turkey

- PREP TIME: 30 m
- COOK TIME: 3 h 30 m
- BRINING TIME: 18 h
- TOTAL TIME: 4 h
- SERVINGS: 12

Fixings

- 10 OUNCES legitimate salt generally 1¼ cups Morton's or 1¾ cups Diamond Crystal
- ¾ CUP dark colored sugar or maple syrup
- Five sprigs of new wise
- 5 sprigs new thyme
- Two huge sprigs of new rosemary
- Four inlet leaves
- Five squashed garlic cloves
- 3 TO 4 dried stew peppers
- 1 TABLESPOON dark peppercorns
- the strip of 2 oranges
- 1 TO 2 GALLONS cold water

- For roasting the turkey:
- 1/2 CUP Butter dissolved.
- 15 POUND Whole Turkey or bigger

Directions

1. Combine the salt, sugar, new herbs, garlic, stew peppers, peppercorns, and orange strip in a pan with around 4 cups of water. Heat to the point of boiling to break down the salt and sugar and afterward expel it from the heat.

2. Cool the saltwater totally and afterward pour the saline solution over the turkey in a brining pack or enormous vessel that will fit into your fridge. Fill the vessel with cold water, so the turkey is secured and refrigerate.

3. Brine turkey for 8 to 18 hours. At that point, expel the turkey from the saline solution and dispose of the saltwater. Flush the turkey well and dry with paper towels. Spot the turkey on a rack in the roasting skillet and refrigerate for a few hours or medium-term to dry.

4. Preheat the oven to 450°F and expel the turkey from the fridge.

5. Do not add season to the turkey again before roasting. Brush liquefied spread on the turkey bosom and legs and stuff crisp herbs and crushed cloves of garlic inside the depression of the turkey. Empty the stock or wine into the base of the roasting skillet and move the turkey to the oven. Roast the turkey, yet begin checking the temperature of the turkey at any rate 30 minutes before you anticipate that it should be done. Treat the turkey with the drippings at regular intervals or thereabouts and add more water to the roasting dish if the dribbling dissipates too rapidly. In the event that the bosom begins to darker too rapidly, essentially tent it with aluminum foil. At the point when the inward temperature of the turkey (taken in the bosom meat, within the thigh and the outside thigh) arrives at 165°F, expel the turkey from the oven and let it lay on the counter, secured freely with aluminum foil for at any rate 30 minutes before cutting.

Potato Gratin

- PREP TIME: 15 m
- COOK TIME: 1 h 15 m
- TOTAL TIME: 1 h 30 m
- SERVINGS:

Fixings

- 2½ CUPS creamer, partitioned

- 2 CLOVES of garlic crushed level
- ½ TEASPOON salt
- freshly ground dark pepper
- ¼ TEASPOON ground nutmeg
- 2 POUNDS potatoes, around 5 or 6, stripped and cut (¼-inch cuts)
- 1 CUP ground Parmesan cheddar
- 1 TABLESPOON margarine, cut into little solid shapes
- fresh thyme leaves discretionary

Guidelines

1. Preheat the oven to 350° F.

2. Combine 1½ cups of creamer with the garlic in a shallow skillet or gratin container and bring it to a stew on the stovetop. Stew for 15 minutes. Season with the salt, pepper, and nutmeg.

3. Turn the heat off underneath the creamer and include the cut potatoes, isolating the cuts and squeezing them into the cream to guarantee they are altogether conveyed equally. Include enough of the staying cream to cover every one of the potatoes simply. Top with the Parmesan cheddar, dab with margarine, and move the dish to the oven.

4. Bake in the oven for 50 to an hour, or until the potatoes are delicate and pleasantly cooked on top. Present with a little crisp thyme on top whenever wanted.

Cranberry Sauce

- PREP TIME: 5 m
- COOK TIME: 20 m
- TOTAL TIME: 25 m
- SERVINGS: 8 2 cups

Fixings

- ½ CUP squeezed orange or water

- ½ CUP of sugar
- 4 CUPS crisp cranberries 1 (12-ounce pack)
- PINCH salt

Discretionary INGREDIENTS

- 1 cinnamon stick
- 2 TABLESPOONS orange pizzazz
- PINCH crisply ground nutmeg

Guidelines

1. Combine the squeezed orange (or water) and sugar in a 2 to 3-quart pan and bring to a stew to break down the sugar. Include the cranberries and cinnamon stick (if utilizing).

2. Simmer delicately for 20 minutes, or until every one of the cranberries has popped and separated into a sauce. Include orange pizzazz and nutmeg (if utilizing).

3. Bring to room temperature before serving.

Mile High Apple Pie

- PREP TIME: 20 m
- COOK TIME: 55 m
- RESTING TIME: 30 m
- TOTAL TIME: 1 h 15 m
- SERVINGS: 8

Fixings

- Basic Pie Dough for 2 9-inch circles
- 9 CUPS stripped cored and cut apples (around 3 pounds; ½-inch cuts)
- 1/3 CUP dark colored sugar
- 1/3 CUP granulated sugar in addition to additional for sprinkling on top

- 1 TEASPOON ground cinnamon
- ¼ TEASPOON ground nutmeg or ideally newly ground nutmeg
- ¼ TEASPOON allspice
- ¼ TEASPOON salt
- 4 TEASPOON cornstarch
- 1 TO 2 TABLESPOONS spread cut into solid shapes
- 1 egg delicately beaten

Directions

1. Preheat the oven to 425°F.

2. Roll out the baked good circles on a floured surface until they are about ¼-inch thick. Spot one hover of turned out batter into the pie dish and delicately press the mixture into the edges of the dish. Trim the edges of the cake and refrigerate the pie shell for 30 minutes. Spot the other hover of the mixture in the cooler, either moving it up in material paper or a silicone heating sheet.

3. Combine the apples, sugars, and flavors in an enormous bowl and hurl together. Allow this to sit and macerate for at any rate 30 minutes. Strain the apples through a colander into a bowl, holding the fluid. Get this fluid to a stew a little pot on the stove and diminish it nearly significantly.

4. Toss the apples with the cornstarch and afterward return the diminished fluid to the blend. Move the apples to the pie dish with the turned out baked good. Heap the apples high in the dish and spot the apples with the margarine. Wrap the staying turned out cake hover over the top.

5. Brush the lower edge of the baked good with water, and seal the top edge of the cake down on the base edge. When fixed together, trim the baked good around the dish. Make 5 or so cuts or patterns in the baked good to allow steam to avoid during cooking. Brush the outside of the pie with the delicately beaten egg, and sprinkle the surface with sugar.

6. Bake in the oven for 30 minutes. Diminish the heat to 350°F and keep on preparing for another 20 to 25 minutes. In the event that anytime the edges of the hull are getting excessively dull, spread the edges with aluminum foil. The pie is done when pleasantly caramelized on top, and the apples inside are delicate and delicate when penetrated with a paring blade through one of the vent cuts.

Fundamental Gravy

- PREP TIME: 5 m
- COOK TIME: 10 m
- TOTAL TIME: 15 m
- SERVINGS: 8 2 cups

Fixings

- 2 TABLESPOON margarine
- 2 TABLESPOON flour
- 2 CUPS stock chicken, hamburger or mushroom, room temperature
- salt and naturally ground dark pepper
- Other discretionary seasonings: soy sauce, Worcestershire sauce, crisp herbs, cream

Guidelines

1. Preheat a 2-quart pan on medium heat.
2. Add margarine and liquefy. Gather flour and whisk margarine and flour into a single unit. Cook, normally blending for 2 minutes.
3. Add 1 cup of stock, whisking constantly.
4. Bring the blend to a bubble and thicken it. Put it in a safe spot.
5. When you have wrapped up your meat, pour the drippings from the roast into a fat separator. Let the fat ascent to the surface and empty the tasty drippings into the sauce. This will weaken the sauce to the correct consistency and include the flavor from the roast to your sauce. If you need the sauce somewhat looser, bit by bit includes the rest of your stock.

Sweet Potato and Fennel Soup

- PREP TIME: 10 m
- COOK TIME: 8 m
- TOTAL TIME: 18 m

- SERVINGS: 6

Fixings

- 2 TABLESPOONS margarine
- 1 TABLESPOON olive oil
- ½ onion slashed (about ½ cup)
- 1½ bulbs fennel slashed
- 3 sweet potatoes stripped and slashed (around 6 cups)
- 4 CUPS water
- ½ TEASPOON salt or more to taste
- freshly ground dark pepper
- 3 TABLESPOONS fennel fronds

Guidelines

1. Preheat the pressure cooker on the BROWN setting.

2. Add the margarine and olive oil and cook the onions and fennel until delicate. Include the sweet potatoes and water and lock the cover set up.

3. Pressure cook on HIGH for 8 minutes.

5. Using a drenching blender, purée the soup until no bumps remain, and the soup is smooth. (Then again, you can utilize a blender or food processor and purée the soup in groups.) Thin the soup with water until you've arrived at the ideal consistency. Include salt and naturally ground dark pepper. Present with a touch of acrid cream and a portion of the fennel fronds to decorate.

Cauliflower Cheddar Soup with Hazelnut Dukkah

- PREP TIME: 15 m
- COOK TIME: 6 m
- TOTAL TIME: 21 m

- SERVINGS: 2

Fixings

- 2 TEASPOONS olive oil
- ½ onion cleaved (½ cup)
- 1 little clove garlic crushed
- ½ TEASPOON new thyme leaves
- ½ medium head of cauliflower hacked (around 4 cups or 1 pound)
- salt and newly ground dark pepper
- 1 CUP chicken stock
- 1 CUP ground sharp white cheddar
- extra virgin olive oil

HAZELNUT DUKKAH

- ¼ CUP hazelnuts
- 2 TABLESPOONS almonds
- 1 TABLESPOON pumpkin seeds
- ½ TEASPOON fennel seeds
- 2 TEASPOONS coriander seeds
- 1 TABLESPOON white sesame seeds
- 2 TEASPOONS cumin seeds
- ½ TEASPOON dried thyme
- 1 TEASPOON paprika
- 1 TABLESPOON dark sesame seeds
- ½ TEASPOON coarse ocean salt

Directions

1. Pre-heat a multi-work 2-quart pressure cooker utilizing the BROWN setting.

2. Add the oil, onion, garlic, and thyme. Cook for 4 to 5 minutes, mixing every so often.

3. Pressure cook on HIGH for 6 minutes.

4. Move the nuts and seeds to a bubble to cool. Include the fennel seeds, coriander seeds, sesame seeds, cumin seeds, and thyme to the skillet and toast until fragrant – around 3 minutes. Move the seeds and herbs to the bowl with the nuts. Let the blend cool for a few minutes and afterward move to a smaller than usual chopper and heartbeat until the blend is brittle, however not a powder. Move the nut and seed blend to bowl and mix in the paprika, dark sesame seeds, and ocean salt.

5. Purée the soup utilizing a blender (recollecting not to fill the blender the greater part full with the hot blend) or a submersion blender. Include the cheddar, and mix until the cheddar has all liquefied.

6. Serve the soup in bowls, shower the additional virgin olive oil on top in any structure you like.

Curried Sweet Potato Soup

- PREP TIME: 10 m
- COOK TIME: 40 m
- TOTAL TIME: 50 m
- SERVINGS: 6

Fixings

- 2 TABLESPOONS margarine
- 1 TABLESPOON olive oil
- ½ onion slashed (about ½ cup)
- 5 TO 6 sweet potatoes stripped and diced
- 1 TABLESPOON curry powder

- 4 CUPS chicken stock vegetable stock or water
- ¾ CUP squeezed orange
- ½ TEASPOON salt or more to taste naturally ground dark pepper
- ½ CUP harsh cream discretionary
- 3 TABLESPOONS slashed crisp parsley

Guidelines

1. Melt the margarine alongside the olive oil in a stockpot or Dutch oven over medium heat. Include the onion and cook for 5 to 7 minutes. The onion ought to be translucent, not dark-colored.

2. Add the sweet potatoes and curry powder, and keep on cooking for another 6 to 8 minutes. Include the chicken stock, vegetable stock, or water and keep on stewing for an additional 20 minutes. Mix in the squeezed orange.

3. Using a blender, food processor, food factory, or submersion blender, puree the soup until no lumps remain, and the soup is smooth. Return the soup to the stovetop and slender the soup with water until you've arrived at the ideal consistency. Include salt and naturally ground dark pepper. Present with a dab of harsh cream and slashed parsley to decorate.

The French & Canadian Yellow Split Pea Soup

- PREP TIME: 15 m
- COOK TIME: 15 m
- PRESSURE RELEASE: 10 m
- TOTAL TIME: 30 m
- SERVINGS: 6

Fixings

- 1 TABLESPOON spread
- 1 onion hacked
- 2 carrots hacked

- 2 CLOVES garlic crushed
- 4 sprigs new thyme
- 2 CUPS yellow split peas
- 1 ham bone or smoked pork pawn flushed (discretionary)
- 12 OUNCES cooked ham cut into huge
- 3-INCH pieces
- 2 inlet leaves
- 6 CUPS water

- ½ CUP sharp cream
- 1 TABLESPOON maple syrup

Guidelines

1. Preheat the pressure cooker is utilizing the BROWN setting.

2. Add the margarine to the pressure cooker and sauté the onion, carrot, garlic, and thyme. Cook until the vegetables simply begin to mollify – around 5 minutes. Include the split peas, ham bone, ham lumps, sound leaves, and the water. Lock the top set up.

3. Pressure cook on HIGH for 10 minutes.

4. While the soup is cooking, join the sharp cream and maple syrup in a little bowl.

5. At that point discharge, any outstanding pressure utilizing the QUICK-RELEASE method and cautiously evacuate the top. Expel the ham sell from the pot and let it sufficiently cool to pull any meat from the bone. Expel the pieces of ham and cut into little bones. Present with a sprinkle or touch of the maple cream on top.

Split Pea Soup - Pressure Cooker Version

- PREP TIME: 10 m

- COOK TIME: 10 m
- RELEASE TIME: 10 m
- TOTAL TIME: 20 m
- SERVINGS:

+

-

Fixings

- 1 TABLESPOON margarine or oil
- 1 onion slashed
- 2 stalks of celery slashed
- 2 carrots slashed
- 2 CLOVES garlic minced
- 4 sprigs crisp thyme
- 2 CUPS dried green or yellow split peas
- 1 ham bone or smoked pork sell flushed
- 6 CUPS water
- salt and naturally ground dark pepper
- 5 OUNCES cooked ham thick cut ham from the store is great
- sour cream and bread garnishes to decorate discretionarily

Directions

1. Preheat the pressure cooker is utilizing the BROWN setting.

2. Add the oil to the pressure cooker and afterward include the onion, celery, and garlic. Cook until the vegetables simply start to mellow. Include the crisp thyme, split peas, ham bone, and the water and lock the top set up.

3. Pressure cook on HIGH for 10 minutes.

4. Let the pressure drop NATURALLY and cautiously expel the cover.

5. Remove the ham pawn from the pot and let it sufficiently cool to pull any meat from the bone. Put the meat in a safe spot.

6. Meanwhile, utilizing a blender, or a submersion blender purée the soup and return it to the pressure cooker. A a little lemon squeeze, and slight the soup with a little water if essential. Return the meat from the ham issue that remains to be worked out cooker, alongside the cooked ham.

7. Serve with some hard bread and a green serving of mixed greens.

Corned Beef with Cabbage, Potatoes and Split Pea Mash - Stovetop Version

- PREP TIME: 10 m
- COOK TIME: 2 h
- TOTAL TIME: 2 h 10 m
- SERVINGS:

Fixings

- 1 3-to 3½-pound corned hamburger brisket
- 4 CUPS hamburger stock
- 1 onion quartered
- 3 CLOVES garlic crushed
- 2 cove leaves
- 10 peppercorns
- 1 cinnamon stick
- 10 coriander seeds
- 2 TEASPOONS darker or yellow mustard seeds
- 8 allspice berries

- 6 cloves
- 1 CUP dried yellow split peas
- cheesecloth or a "pudding pack."
- One little to medium head cabbage cut into 6 wedges
- 6 enormous carrots cut into huge pieces
- 6 medium white potatoes split
- 2 TABLESPOONS spread
- salt and newly ground dark pepper

Directions

1. Rinse the corned meat brisket and spot it in a huge stockpot. Spread with meat stock and include the onion, garlic, and flavors to the pot. (On the off chance that your corned hamburger accompanies a flavoring parcel, you do have the alternative of utilizing that rather than the flavors recorded here.) Place the dried split peas into a pudding pack, or envelop them by the cheesecloth, tying the cheesecloth freely with the goal that the peas have space to grow. Push the pack down into the fluid, including a cup or two of water, to ensure everything is submerged. Spread the pot with a top and carry everything to a stew. Lower the heat and stew for 1 hour and 30 minutes.

2. Add the cabbage wedges, carrots and potatoes, return the cover and keep on stewing for 30 minutes.

3. When every one of the vegetables is delicate, move the cooked split peas to a bowl. Expel the cheesecloth and dispose of it. Squash the peas with a wooden spoon, mixing in the margarine and season with salt and bunches of crisply ground dark pepper.

4. Slice the meat, move then cuts to a huge platter with the vegetables, and serve the crushed, split peas as an afterthought.

Air Fryer Roasted Chestnuts

- PREP TIME: 10 m
- COOK TIME: 15 m
- TOTAL TIME: 25 m

Fixings

- 1 POUND crude chestnuts
- salt discretionary
- oil discretionary

Directions

1. Place the chestnuts level side down on a cutting board. Utilizing a sharp or serrated blade, score the chestnuts, making a point to go right through the shell.

2. Preheat the air fryer to 380ºF.

3. Place the scored chestnuts in the air fryer container, scored side up. Air-fry at 380ºF for 15 minutes or until the shells have stripped move in the opposite direction from the nuts. Expel the nuts from the air fryer and let them sufficiently cool to have the option to deal with them.

4. Peel the shells off the chestnuts and dispose of. Utilize a paring blade to strip away the light darker skin to uncover the yellow nut.

5. Use the chestnuts entire in appetizing braised chicken dishes, hack them up to use in stuffings and dressings, or puree to use in sweet preparing recipes or to make a chestnut cream.

Air Fried Beer Battered Fish

- PREP TIME: 10 m
- COOK TIME: 12 m
- RESTING TIME: 20 m
- TOTAL TIME: 42 m
- SERVINGS: 4

Fixings

- 1 CUP generally useful flour
- 2 TABLESPOONS cornstarch
- ½ TEASPOON preparing pop

- 6 OUNCES brew
- 1 egg beaten
- ¾ CUP generally useful flour
- ½ TEASPOON paprika
- 1 TEASPOON salt
- ¼ TEASPOON crisply ground dark pepper.

Guidelines

1. Combine the flour, cornstarch, and heating soft drink in an enormous bowl. Include the brew and egg and mix until smooth. Spread the bowl of a hitter with saran wrap and refrigerate for in any event 20 minutes.

2. Combine the flour, paprika, salt, dark pepper, and cayenne pepper in a shallow digging container.

3. Pat the codfish filets dry with a paper towel. Plunge the fish into the player, covering all sides. Let the abundance player trickle off and afterward cover each filet with the prepared flour. Sprinkle any extra flour on the fish filets and pat delicately to stick the flour to the hitter.

4. Preheat the air fryer to 390°F.

5. Generously spritz the two sides of the covered fish filets with vegetable oil and spot them in the air fryer container. Air-fry for 12 minutes at 390ºF. Spritz with more oil during the cooking procedure if there are any dry spots on the covering.

6. Serve quickly with lemon wedges, malt vinegar, and tartar sauce. It's ideal with some air-fried French fries and coleslaw as well!

Turkey, Mushroom and Broccoli Calzone

- PREP TIME: 20 m
- COOK TIME: 30 m
- RESTING TIME: 10 m
- TOTAL TIME: 1 h

- SERVINGS:

4

Fixings

- 1½ CUPS broccoli florets cut into pieces
- olive oil
- 8 OUNCES mushrooms cut
- 1½ CUPS cooked turkey bosom cut into ½-inch blocks
- 1 CUP ground mozzarella cheddar
- 1¼ CUPS ricotta cheddar
- ½ TEASPOON Italian flavoring
- ½ TEASPOON salt
- freshly ground dark pepper
- 16-OUNCES natively constructed or locally acquired pizza mixture
- 2 TABLESPOONS olive oil
- pizza or marinara sauce discretionary

Directions

1. Use a medium pot of water to a bubble and whiten the broccoli in the water for 3 to 4 minutes. Channel and run the broccoli under virus water to stop the cooking procedure and put the broccoli in a safe spot.

2. Preheat a sauté dish over medium-high heat. Include a little olive oil and sauté the mushrooms until seared.

3. Preheat a pizza stone, pizza steel, or overwhelming preparing sheet in the oven at 400°F for 20 to 30 minutes.

4. Combine the turkey, mozzarella cheddar, ricotta cheddar, Italian flavoring, salt, and crisply ground dark pepper in a bowl. Overlay the whitened broccoli and sautéed mushrooms into the blend.

5. Divide the pizza batter down the middle. Stretch or fold one portion of the mixture into a 10-inch circle. The spread portion of the turkey and cheddar blend on one portion of the hover of the mixture, leaving around one inch of batter void around the edge.

6. Fold the other portion of the batter over the cheddar blend, nearly to the edge of the mixture to frame a half-moon. Overlay the base edge of the batter up the ludicrous edge and crease the mixture around the edges to make the outside layer and seal the calzone shut. Brush the mixture with olive oil. Rehash with the rest of the part of the pizza mixture to make the second calzone.

7. Place the calzones on a pizza strip fixed with material paper. (If you don't have a pizza strip, utilize a turned over-preparing sheet fixed with material paper.) With a snappy, simple, and certain sliding movement (as if you were pulling a tablecloth off a table without upsetting what was on top!) slide the calzones alongside the material paper to the preheated pizza stone or preparing sheet in the oven. (The material paper should slide off with the calzones, yet don't stress – the material will dark-colored; however, it won't burst into flames.)

8. Remove the calzones from the oven utilizing the pizza strip and let them cool for 10 minutes before serving. Present with pizza sauce as an afterthought, whenever wanted.

Chicken-Paillard with Burrata and Roasted Cherry Tomatoes

- PREP TIME: 20 m
- COOK TIME: 10 m
- TOTAL TIME: 30 m
- SERVINGS: 2

Fixings

- 2 5-ounce boneless skinless chicken bosoms
- 2 TABLESPOONS flour
- salt and newly ground dark pepper
- 1 egg beaten
- 1¼ CUPS panko bread pieces
- olive oil

- 1 CUP cherry tomatoes
- juice of half of a lemon
- 4 CUPS child arugula
- 6 OUNCES burrata

Directions

1. Spot it on a cutting board and lay the palm of your hand level over the chicken. Hold a sharp blade corresponding to the slicing board and cut through the chicken, preventing around one inch from the opposite side of the bosom. Open the chicken bosom like a "book." Spot a bit of saran wrap over the chicken and pound the bosom with the level side of a meat hammer or moving pin until it is an even thickness - about ½ inch thick.

2. Set up a digging station with 3 shallow skillets. Spot flour in the principal container and season with salt and dark pepper. Beat the egg in a subsequent dish. Pour the panko bread morsels in the third dish and season with salt and pepper.

3. Dredge the two sides of the chicken in the flour, at that point plunge into the egg, and afterward cover the chicken bosom with the panko bread pieces. Tenderly pat to stick the scraps to the chicken bosom.

4. Heat the olive oil in a huge skillet over medium-high heat. Spot the breaded chicken paillard in the container and cook for around 2 to 3 minutes on each side, until the chicken is carmelized and cooked through.

5. Transfer the chicken to a plate. Add the cherry tomatoes and sauté for a couple of moments on high heat until they begin to dark-colored and burst somewhat. Season with salt and pepper.

6. crisp lemon squeeze, salt, and dark pepper.

7. Place the chicken paillard on a serving dish, top with arugula and some cherry tomatoes and dab spoonfuls of the burrata on or by the chicken. Present with some broke dark pepper.

Sprouting Onion

- PREP TIME: 15 m
- COOK TIME: 25 m
- TOTAL TIME: 40 m

- SERVINGS: 4

Fixings

- 1 huge Vidalia onion stripped
- 2 eggs
- ½ CUP milk
- 1 CUP flour
- 1 TEASPOON salt
- ½ TEASPOON dark pepper
- ¼ TEASPOON cayenne pepper
- ½ TEASPOON paprika
- ½ TEASPOON garlic powder

Plunging SAUCE:

- ½ CUP mayonnaise
- ½ CUP ketchup
- 1 TEASPOON Worcestershire sauce
- ½ TEASPOON cayenne pepper
- ½ TEASPOON paprika
- ½ TEASPOON onion powder

Guidelines

1. Spot the now level, stem end of the onion down on a cutting board with the root end looking up. Make 16 cuts around the onion, beginning with your blade tip ½-inch away from the root, so you never cut through the root. Start by making cuts at 12, 3, 6, and 9 o'clock around the onion. At that point, make three cuts down the onion in the middle of every one of the first four cuts. Turn onion over, delicately separate the onion petals, and expel the free bits of onion in the middle.

2. In a subsequent bowl, consolidate the flour, salt, dark pepper, cayenne pepper, paprika, and garlic powder.

3. Preheat the air fryer to 350°F.

4. Sprinkle the flour blend everywhere throughout the onion to cover it and get in the middle of the onion petals. Surrender the onion to shake off the abundance flour deliberately and afterward move the onion to the vacant flour bowl, again cut side up.

5. Pour the egg blend everywhere throughout the onion to cover all the flour. Let it drench for a moment in the blend. Cautiously expel the onion, tipping it topsy turvy to deplete off any overabundance egg, and move it to the unfilled egg bowl, again cut side up.

6. Finally, sprinkle the flour blend over the onion a subsequent time, ensuring the onion is very much covered, and every one of the petals has the prepared flour blend on them. Cautiously turn the onion over, shake off any abundance flour and move it to a plate or preparing sheet. Splash the onion liberally with vegetable oil.

7. Transfer the onion, slice side up to the air fryer bushel, and air-fry for 25 minutes. The onion petals will open all the more completely as it cooks, so shower with increasingly vegetable oil in any event twice during the cooking time.

8. While the onion is cooking, make the plunging sauce by consolidating all the plunge fixings and blending admirably. Serve the Blooming Onion when it leaves the air fryer with plunging sauce as an afterthought.

Air-Fried Salt and Pepper Shrimp

- PREP TIME: 20 m
- COOK TIME: 30 m
- TOTAL TIME: 50 m
- SERVINGS: 6

Fixings

- 1 CUP generally useful flour
- ½ CUP cornstarch
- 2 TEASPOONS salt
- 2 TEASPOONS coarsely ground dark pepper

- 1 POUND extra-huge shrimp stripped and deveined with tails left on
- 2 eggs
- canola or vegetable oil
- 1 TEASPOON olive oil
- 2 CLOVES garlic daintily cut
- 1 INCH ginger daintily cut
- 4 cherry peppers cut
- 3 scallions cleaved

Guidelines

1. Set up a digging station. Join the flour, cornstarch, salt, and dark pepper and gap the blend between two zipper sealable plastic packs. Beat the eggs together in a bowl. Add the shrimp to one sack of flour and shake them around to cover. Working in bunches, expel the shrimp from the pack of flour, shaking off any overabundance and dunk each shrimp in the beaten eggs before setting them in the second sack of flour and shaking to cover once more. Put the covered shrimp in a safe spot.

2. Pre-heat air fryer to 400°F.

3. Transfer the covered shrimp to the air fryer crate and spritz liberally with oil.

4. Air-fry, the shrimp in groups for 6 minutes.

5. Include the garlic, ginger and cherry peppers and sauté for three minutes, until the peppers have relaxed somewhat.

6. When the last bunch of shrimp has got done with cooking.

Herbed Sourdough Croutons

- PREP TIME: 10 m
- COOK TIME: 7 m
- TOTAL TIME: 17 m
- SERVINGS: 8

Fixings

- 4 CUPS cubed sourdough bread 1-inch 3D shapes (around 8 ounces)
- 1 TABLESPOON olive oil
- 1 TEASPOON new thyme leaves
- ¼ - ½ TEASPOON salt
- freshly ground dark pepper

Directions

1. Combine all fixings in a bowl and taste to ensure it is prepared exactly as you would prefer.
2. Pre-heat the air fryer to 400°F for 2 minutes.
3. Toss the bread 3D shapes into the air fryer and air-fry for 5 to 7 minutes, shaking the container more than once while they cook.
4. Serve warm or store in an airtight compartment.

Sheet Pan Fish and Chips - Oven Version

- PREP TIME: 10 m
- COOK TIME: 40 m
- TOTAL TIME: 50 m
- SERVINGS: 4

Fixings

- 3 Russet potatoes huge stripped cut into ½-inch sticks
- canola oil
- seasoned salt
- ¼ CUP generally useful flour
- 2 TABLESPOONS Dijon mustard

- 2 eggs
- ¾ CUP prepared breadcrumbs
- 1 lemon zested
- 4 lemon cut into wedges

Directions

1. Soakand strain the potatoes and pat them dry with a perfect kitchen towel.
2. Preheat the oven to 450°F.
3. Toss the potato sticks with some canola oil and a sprinkling of prepared salt, place them on an enormous 12-inch by 17-inch sheet skillet in a solitary layer and move the dish to the oven. Prepare at 450°F for 25 minutes.
4. Add the flour to the primary shallow dish. In a subsequent dish, whisk the Dijon mustard and eggs together. In the third dish, join the breadcrumbs, lemon get-up-and-go, paprika, and salt. Dig the pieces of fish in the flour first. At that point, dunk them into the egg blend, allowing any overabundance to dribble off, lastly cover them with the breadcrumb blend. Pat the breadcrumbs on delicately to ensure the morsels hold fast to the fish.
5. After 25 minutes of preparing time, expel the dish from the oven and turn the potatoes over, pushing them to the other side of the sheet container. Spritz the covered fish filets liberally with canola oil on all sides and add them to the sweet dish. Prepare at 450°F for 15 minutes. The fish ought to be crispy on top and flaky within.
6. Serve the fish sticks and french fries with malt vinegar, tartar sauce and lemon wedges, and a little coleslaw as an afterthought.

Raspberry Almond Fruit Squares - Oven Version

- PREP TIME: 20 m
- COOK TIME: 45 m
- TOTAL TIME: 1 h 5 m
- SERVINGS: 24

Fixings

- ½ CUP almond glue around 5 ounces

- ¾ CUP unsalted margarine room temperature
- 1 CUP sugar
- 1 egg
- 2 CUPS universally handy flour
- ½ TEASPOON heating powder
- ½ TEASPOON heating pop
- ¼ TEASPOON salt
- 1 CUP seedless raspberry jam
- 4 CUPS raspberries

Morsel TOPPING LAYER:

- ¾ CUP universally handy flour
- ¾ CUP cereal
- ¾ CUP darker sugar
- ¾ CUP cut almonds
- ½ CUP margarine dissolved.

Guidelines

1. Preheat the oven to 350°F. Spot a 15-inch long bit of material paper in a 9-inch by 13-inch heating dish, so the closures reach out over the sides of the container.

2. Combine the almond glue and spread in a food processor, and heartbeat until joined. Include the sugar and egg and procedure until the blend is smooth. Include the flour, preparing powder, heating pop, and salt. Procedure until the batter meets up. Press the blend into the base of the readied preparing container.

3. Whisk the jam until it is smooth. Delicately overlay in the raspberries to cover them with the jam and spoon the raspberry filling over the outside layer.

4. Make the scrap besting. Consolidate the flour, cereal, darker sugar, and almonds in a bowl and hurl to join. Pour the liquefied spread on top and mix the fixings with a fork to shape

coarse disintegrates. Sprinkle the morsel beating over the natural product filling. Move the skillet to the oven.

5. Bake it at the 350ºF for 40 to 45 minutes, until the top is light dark-colored. Expel the container from the oven and let it cool totally on a wire rack. Lift the material paper to evacuate the heated raspberry and almond out of the skillet and move it to a cutting board. Slice into 20 to 24 squares.

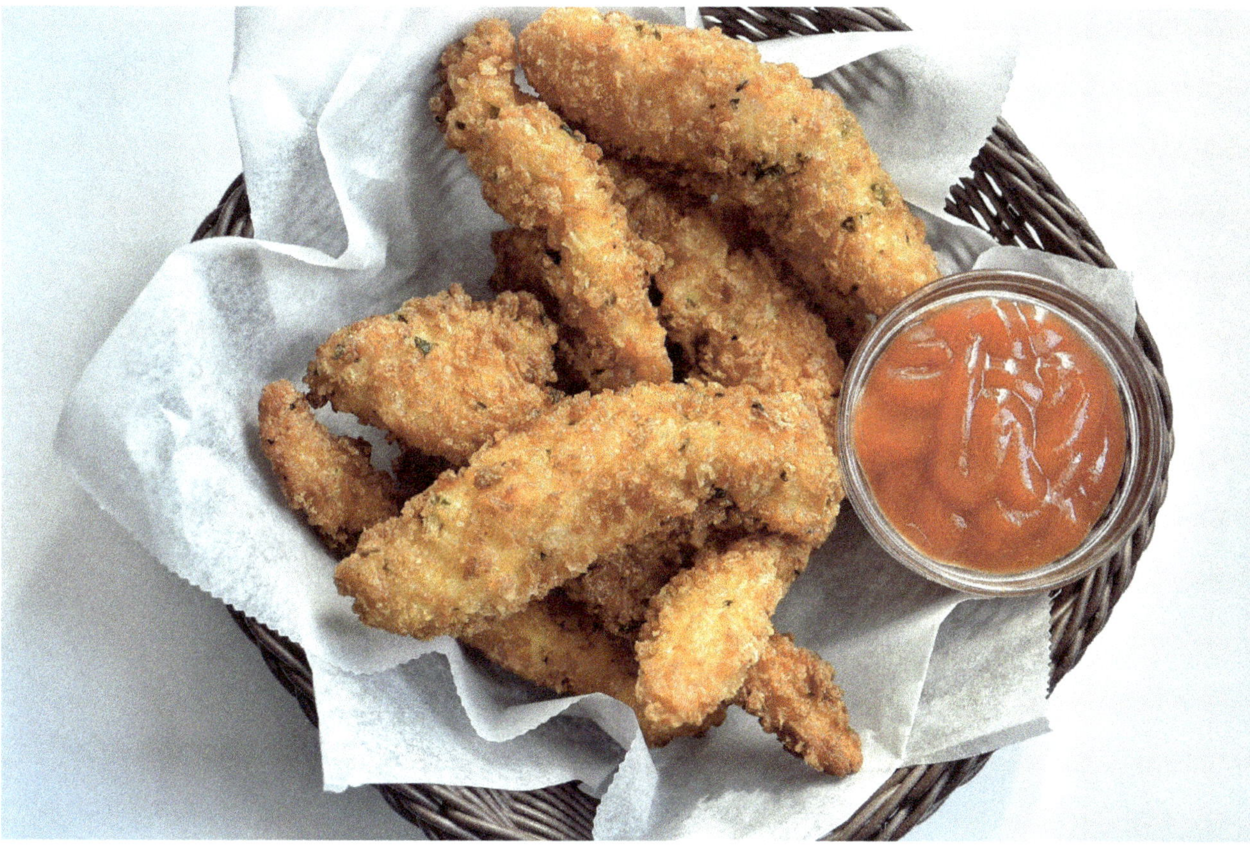

CPSIA information can be obtained
at www.ICGtesting.com
Printed in the USA
LVHW061932250521
688474LV00003B/608

9 781667 100234